THE TIME FOR
FREEDOM

CHANGING THE WAY WE SEE THINGS NOW

ELAINE MACE

Words from If I Were Brave and Butterfly, by Jana Stanfield / Joyce Rouse, used with permission.

Author's photograph by Lesley Burns. Photographer www.sniperphotography.co.uk.

Edited by Clare Christian and Kevin Bermingham

Book interior design and typesetting by Pedernales Publishing, LLC.

Front cover design by Pedernales Publishing, LLC.

British Library Cataloguing in Publication Data.

A catalogue record for this book is available from the British Library.

Paperback edition
ISBN 978-1-908101-31-0

Praise for

The Time For Freedom
Changing the Way We See Things Now
by Elaine Mace

'Elaine Mace is a passionate and inspiring woman. She has demonstrated the power of living with purpose and the ability to work with others to help them find their goals. Elaine will stay with you as you learn and offer unconditional support as well as loving challenges. I wish her well with The Time for Freedom – it has an important message for many of us.'

Kate Howe, Workshop participant

'The energy Elaine brings to her work with people is highly motivating and truly inspiring. Her perception and insight support people in creating huge steps forward and I find her an absolute joy to be with.'

Steve Barnes, Facilitator and Coach

'Elaine provides an exceptional level of professional insight and dedication, personal warmth and integrity to everything she does. She is perceptive and analytical of situations and management matters as well as being a constructive and inspiring coach. She loves life and values relationships. Always constructive and positive in her feedback, Elaine's glass is always full – never mind half full!'

Jeanette Redding, School Improvement Adviser

'Having got to know Elaine, firstly as her Dru Yoga teacher and mentor, and then as her friend, one of her great qualities is that she loves people. She takes a genuine interest in their lives. She will always find a way to help someone discover their strengths and stand in their power. In the famous words of Louis Pasteur, "Let me tell you the secret that has led me to my goal: my strength lies solely in my tenacity." Elaine has the same such tenacity. She really cares.'

Shona Sutherland, Dru Yoga Teacher Trainer

'I have been privileged to be with Elaine and have always been struck by her enthusiasm, passion and insight … her sense of purpose about helping others is a delightful assault on the senses and she leaves others feeling motivated and enlightened with a clear understanding of their 'what next' which allows them to confidently take the next steps on life's journey'

Dave Jessop, Peak Performance Coach

'Elaine brings her depth of understanding, her commitment to growth and development, her insight and intuition, her clarity and creativity into everything she does – and she does it with kindness, love and empathy in a straight talking way. Working with Elaine is like a breath of fresh air and she creates magic along the way.'

Teresa Garfield, Coach, facilitator, and trainer

'I have had the privilege of seeing Elaine in action both delivering Goal Mapping and living her own life through using her own Goal Map. She is a warm and wonderfully inspiring person with the gift of letting you feel that you are the most important person to her in the moment. She always makes time, is passionate about helping others and in a world of "take, take, take" she is all "give, give, give". More people like Elaine please.'

Richard Gilbert, Equilibrium Network Limited

This book is dedicated to anyone and everyone who has ever found loving, trusting and believing in themselves to be a challenge.

ACKNOWLEDGEMENTS

Thank you for taking this book from the shelf and reading it. Although I wrote *The Time for Freedom,* and much of my own story guided what I wrote, yet I feel that it has been a team effort.

I want to thank my wonderful, gorgeous Team of Wings who with their love, honesty, and proofreading skills have helped me to find my wings and soar.

I want to thank Kate Howe, Marysia Appleton, Soryl Angel, Pauline Cargill, Chris Wade, Cecile Buxton, Jackie Wallace, Tony Wiseman, Pam Hall, Richard Gilbert, Caroline Argent, Carole Murphy, Gay Jacobsen, Mari Bruce and Maggie Parker. I also want to acknowledge my special friend Debra Poulson who shared her intuitive sparkle.

Thank you to my mentor and publisher Kevin Bermingham of 90 Day Books, without whom *The Time for Freedom* would still be a thought.

Thank you to my amazing son Maximilian Xamonakis, who shone his light when I needed it the most. And to David James who shared his wisdom, and patience and unconditionally supported me each time I lost myself in my *Time for Freedom* world.

Everyone gave me little gem-sized pieces of the puzzle, which when pieced together, have supported me in creating the whole of *The Time for Freedom*. I could not have written this without you.

Thank you

Contents

FOREWORD by SANGEETA MAYNE

"How does one become a butterfly?" she asked "You must want to fly so much that you are willing to give up being a caterpillar" she replied.

Hope for the flowers, by Trina Paulus

As we transcend the various stages of our lives and move into new chapters, there is always that point in between where we must let go of what has been, so that we are free to move to what can be. Sometimes we do this completely unaware of the process, often propelling ourselves into new pastures, only to realise later that we and life have changed.

And sometimes we find that unless we can let go we are unable to move forwards with any great authenticity. Desire for what we want, hope and dream about next is not enough. It must be matched by a desire, willingness and acceptance to let go of who we have become thus far and of life as we currently know it.

This book describes Elaine Mace's incredible journey of reaching this place at a very poignant time in her life. She describes her journey of achieving a place of willingness to give up being a caterpillar, her wake up call, her trials and tribulations, her joys and revelations, as she spreads her wings to fly as a beautiful butterfly. Her story is full of courage, inspiration and hope for anyone faced with the reality that life has more to give.

The *MACE* Pathway guides us step by step through the innermost journey we must take to live life to the full. It is packed with practical viewpoints, exercises, tips and guidelines to engage all our senses, to enliven our mind, body and spirit and to move us into forward action at any age.

In a world where we now live longer than at any other time in our history, with the average age for retirement in the UK continually increasing for both men and women, this book will have you ask the fundamental question, "Just how old is too old for me now?"

BEGINNING THOUGHTS for the READER

'A journey of a lifetime,
over a couple of
moves into realising
her own special
gifts.'

Debra Poulson, artist

Dear Reader,

I got a 'life' wake up call and I wanted to hit the snooze button, but I didn't.

I believe this happened so that I wouldn't get too comfortable, fall asleep, and miss the rest of my life.

This book is about doing the things you need to do that make you feel good about yourself, so that you change the way you see things now. I want this book to catapult you out of your present situation and into the centre of your dreams. I want this book to give you the leg up you need to get you over your wall so you can create movement, action, creativity, and enjoyment in your life. I believe that we are all born on this earth to make a difference, wherever we find ourselves and giving up on ourselves is not an option, particularly in mid-life.

The Time for Freedom is not a 'how to' book or even a 'how not to' book. It is a book about living your best life in middle age, your time for freedom. I invite you to read this book, which is a rich mix of universal laws, ancient thoughts and truths, shared ideas, practical techniques, personal stories, quotes, musings and prompts, to support you in unearthing your buried dreams.

I was employed as a full time teacher for over thirty years. In 2011, I left teaching and now I speak regularly to audiences all over the UK. I create and run workshops for children, young people and adults as well as offering one to one coaching. Drawing on my life's experiences, skills, understanding and knowledge I have written *The Time for Freedom*, which introduces you to The MACE Pathway. It is a simple yet effective structure:

- **M**e – focusing on ourselves first.
- **A**ttitude – considering our attitude.
- **C**ommitment – taking action.
- **E**njoyment – making sure you have fun along the way.

My aim when writing this book has been to inspire you to live a rich and fulfilling life, to view your current situation as an opportunity, and to empower you to change the way you see things now. Mid-life can throw up many questions. There are often major events occurring in life that give us the chance to re-evaluate our situation. Those events might be children leaving home, divorce, loss of interest in work, caring for aged parents, marriage, moving, retirement, depression, work overload, trauma and of course there are many more. If we are working it is not unusual to think that we will put ourselves 'on hold' as retirement is a matter of years away. What we forget is while we are 'on hold' time is not standing still. And, if we changed the way we saw things, there may be an opportunity to have whatever we dream of, or have dreamt of in our lives.

You are a special human being with unique gifts that you share with everyone in your life. Your loved ones, family, friends, colleagues, neighbours, members of your community and acquaintances are all honoured and privileged to know you. We can fall asleep or get lost in our lives. We can forget that we are amazing and can step into lives that aren't ours, or we can make choices that aren't nourishing, or we can dance out of step with the wrong career, friends or partner.

The Time for Freedom is a book about what motivated, inspired and empowered me during my mid-life: what made me leave a secure place of work, take risks, make mistakes and learn to change the way I saw things, so that I could have a creative, fun, relaxed, bold, remarkable and special kind of life.

I hope it will help you do the same.

Best Wishes

Elaine Mace

HOW THIS BOOK WORKS

The Time for Freedom is divided into six chapters. Each chapter is made up of relevant text, personal testimony and stories. The use of stories is a hallmark of *The Time for Freedom*; the stories are designed purposefully to give you examples of human experience and endeavour, and an opportunity to share in another's experience of life. My personal story towards my retirement and the issues and questions that it raised, is woven throughout *The Time for Freedom*. To support me as I moved towards my freedom, I created The MACE Pathway – a structure that I used to explore where I was, where I wanted to go in my life and to change the way I saw things. *The Time for Freedom* introduces you to The MACE Pathway, empowering and inspiring you to change the way you see things now so that you can live your best life.

Pathway Gems

At the end of each chapter there is a section called Pathway Gems. Pathway Gems is a special place where you will find various ideas, practices and suggestions, all to support you towards movement, action, creativity, and enjoyment in your life. Pathway Gems are there for you to digest at your leisure. Having read a chapter, Pathway Gems give you an opportunity to take some time to reflect and acknowledge the amazing person that you are. It is a chance for you to come out and play, to blow the dust off and unearth some of your own hidden gems.

Pathway Gems always begins with Captured Thoughts. These are inspirational, provocative or poignant quotes, for example:

Captured Thoughts

'Our deepest fear is not that we are inadequate. Our deepest fear is that we are powerful beyond measure. It is our light, not our darkness that most frightens us. We ask ourselves, Who am I to be brilliant, gorgeous, talented, and fabulous? Actually who are you not to be?'

Marianne Williams, Author

If you like a Captured Thought, or if it should resonate with you, why not copy it onto card and stick it up in a central place for yourself. You could also meditate on the quote and what it means for you, make a note of it in your journal, or read it to yourself throughout your day. Finding out about the author of the quote and any other of their hidden gems, could also be interesting.

There are four further sections in Pathway Gems: **Movement, Action, Creativity and Enjoyment** and each section includes the following:

Movement. In this section I include movement, activations and examples of Dru Yoga. I am a Dru Yoga and Meditation teacher and I have included in this section of Pathway Gems, some examples of Dru Yoga. 'Dru' translates from Sanskrit as the 'still point'; the still centre of the turning wheel; the calm in the eye of the storm; a state of being in the world but unaffected by its turmoil. Dru Yoga offers practical methods to achieve stillness in motion and is a synthesis of ancient methods, which are now being presented in a modern world, offering a unique perspective on yoga practice.

Guidelines for Movement. It is best to wear loose clothing that allows you to move freely and to use a non-slip mat. It is also best to wait at least two hours after a meal before doing yoga. Make sure that you drink plenty of water after your session. If you have any health issues/ problems, please seek medical advice from a qualified practitioner.

An example of Movement

Movement – Use Activations

Using activations to move our bodies is both nourishing and stimulating. Activations warm our bodies up and prepares them for movement – start slowly and gradually build up the momentum, allowing your body to warm up at its own rhythm and pace. Repeat each exercise until you feel your body loosening.

Arm swings: Stand with your feet hip-width apart and move your arms forwards and backwards. Bend your knees as your arms swing down and straighten them as they swing up. Continue in this way, breathing in as you reach upwards and out as you bend forwards and down.

Gradually increase the swing until your arms reach overhead on the upward swing and finish with your arms swinging up behind you at the end of the downward swing. Try to keep your joints loose.

Action. At various points in each of the chapters in *The Time For Freedom* I make reference to strategies that you could use to extend what I have written about. In the Action section of Pathway Gems I have included practical opportunities to support you in extending the content of the chapter you have just read. I invite you to work through them slowly, and recommend that you record your own discoveries and reflections in your journal.

Also in Action I have included concentration and meditation opportunities. When preparing Action of a quiet nature, choose a place where there are no loud sounds and where no one will disturb you. Make yourself comfortable. Sit rather than lie down and support yourself by training your mind that you have a regular appointment with yourself at the same time each day.

An example of Action

Action - Create a Vision Board

A Life Purpose vision board is a poster board on which you should paste a collage of images that resonate deeply with who you are and ideas about what you want to create in this world. When you start assembling pictures that appeal to this deep self, you unleash one of the most powerful forces on our planet: human imagination. Virtually everything humans use, do, or make, exists because someone thought it up. Sparking your incredibly powerful creative faculty is the reason you make a vision board. The board itself doesn't impact reality; what changes your life is the process of creating the images – combinations of objects and events that will stick in your subconscious mind and steer your choices toward making the vision real.

Vision Board resources:

- Poster board
- A big stack of different magazines
- Glue

Before I began my vision board I carried out a short ritual; I lit a candle and I sat quietly and closed my eyes. I thought kind and open thoughts about myself. I put on soft music. I quietly set my intent, which was to find my Purpose.

Vision Board Steps

- **Step 1**: Go through your magazines and tear the images from them. No gluing yet! Just let yourself have lots of fun looking through magazines and pulling out pictures or words or headlines that strike you as resonating with your Purpose. Have fun with it. Make a big pile of images and phrases and words.

- **Step 2**: Go through the images and begin to lay your favourites on the board. Ask yourself what does this image mean to me? Most likely you'll know the answer. If you don't, but you still love the image, then put it on your vision board anyway. It will have an answer for you soon enough. Eliminate any images that no longer feel right. This step is where your intuition comes in. As you lay the pictures on the board, you'll get a sense how the board should be laid out and this is the start of the evolution of your Purpose.

- **Step 3**: Glue everything onto the board. Add writing if you want. You can paint on it, or write words with markers.

- **Step 4**: If you like you can leave a space for a fantastic photo of yourself.

- **Step 5**: Hang your vision board in a place where you will see it often.

Creativity. Your creativity is an immense force that is inside you. No other person has the special blend of ideas, attitude and perceptions as you. No matter how grumpy lumpy or bumpy you feel your creativity is of value. Crack the shell of your grumps, lumps, and bumps and out will pour your creative treasures. Creativity includes prompts called capturing your whispers. They can act as reminders or nudges for your writing, drawing, painting, or doodling.

An example of Creativity

Creativity – capture your whispers

I invite you to use all, or some of these prompts and record in whatever creative way that you choose.

- When do you feel free?

- What do you feel stands in the way of your achieving some times of personal freedom?

Enjoyment is about having fun along the way. Not worrying about what others may think, feel, say or do. It is about your nourishment. Do what you need to do today to bring Enjoyment into your life.

Keeping a Journal

The dreams and gems you unearth along your pathway need a place for collection. A great way to store and reflect on all those things that have happened in your life is to keep a journal where you can keep track of and record your experiences and your story.

I have two journals: one is by my bedside and is the home of my thoughts, feelings, reflections, loves, passions, musings and my Morning Pages. Morning Pages is a concept devised by Juiia Cameron. She considers that writing Morning Pages is one of two pivotal tools for creative recovery, the other being the artist date. Cameron suggests that in order to retrieve creativity we need to find it and she suggests that we do this through the process that she calls Morning Pages. My second journal is with me always. I write, draw, doodle, and sketch whatever feels right for me in either of my journals.

I have talked to people on my workshops about keeping a journal and sometimes I have found that they resist this because they think they aren't good enough writers, that someone will read their innermost thoughts or that they have much more important things to do. I used to think in that way but I changed my point of view when I stopped thinking of it as a diary, a book in which you write down the day's events. I began to think of it as a container for self-reflection, self-expression, and self-exploration. Retelling the day's events is less relevant than the act of expressing your thoughts, and writing down reflections about events experienced each day. This is an invaluable way to evaluate your performance, set higher standards of excellence, and find new ways to solve difficult problems.

For your journal, I always suggest a notebook that you love. You will know when you've found the right kind of notebook or paper when it makes you swoon and begs to be filled up with your recordings. Whether it is the feel of the paper when it has words written on it, or its smell, or the cover or the messages within. Choose your notebook carefully. Write from your heart.

Paper needs ink and I like to see and feel how the ink moves on the paper. New creative tools are fun. I will use blue, black, pink, green pens. I write big and I write small. I write using all upper case and/or all lower case. This place is for you, so design it for yourself. There's nothing like putting pen to paper to instil you with a sense of optimism, anticipation and excitement about your goals and aspirations. The act of writing something down always makes it more real and more concrete than merely thinking it. When you commit to writing down your thoughts and experiences you have put them into a solid form. I believe there are many benefits to keeping a journal.

- **Knowing yourself better.** Writing can help clarify your thoughts, your emotions, and your reactions to certain people or situations. In addition, as you read back through past journals, you'll have ample evidence of the things that make you happy and those that don't. Journaling is a great tool for self-discovery that will help you build self-confidence and self-knowledge. While writing in your journal you will find yourself identifying the values for which you stand. You will also get to know your processes; how you think, learn, create and use intuition.

- **Capturing your life's story.** A journal is a catalogue of your memories. Over time, your memories become an irreplaceable treasure that can be looked at years from now, by you, or, if you wish, by others. By journaling you will capture not only your life, but also the lives of all the people that surround you. You are creating a record, and with that record in hand it is easier to see the patterns, changes, and shifts in your life.

- **Reducing stress.** Writing in your journal means that you don't carry as much of what you have written about within you. It is on the paper or in the computer. By journaling, you give yourself a powerful form of self-expression, and through that expression you can gain clarity, release, and relief. You will feel calmer and spiritually at ease after a journal writing session.

- **Enhancing intuition and creativity.** While writing in the pages of your journal you will find your inner voice awakening. Journaling will help you in the interpretation of your symbols and dreams, and can increase your memory of events.

- **Strengthening relationships.** Writing about people you know will help you to understand them better and put you in touch with your own feelings about them.

- **Better organisational skills.** By structuring yourself to write regularly, you automatically develop stronger organisational skills, such as list making and time management. Also journaling your goals and what you want to accomplish in your life is an excellent tool to help you get those things done. You can even create a personal checklist of 'things to do'. Through journaling, you can actually see and better understand what you want. E.g. what is important to you, and how you feel? And after organising your thoughts you can create goals and resolutions to support what you are thinking and writing about.

- **Better focus.** While writing in a journal you create more awareness, and therefore more focus on the issues that are important to you. The routine and habit of journaling means making time for yourself, and, when you set aside time for yourself, you can feel the benefit and gain from doing something specifically for yourself. When you're busy and stressed with a mind full of disconnected thoughts flitting here and there, writing about the event or issue will help bring focus and clarity. It will also help you decide on which action to take, or option to choose.

- **Better solutions for your problems.** Writing about problems gives the right side of your brain food for creative problem solving. It's amazing what happens when the creative part of your nature starts working on a problem. You'll soon find solutions bubbling up from your subconscious mind.

- **Personal growth.** Journaling is a vehicle for expressing and creating. It will improve balance and wellbeing and bring you closer to the authentic you.

WELCOME

I was fifty-eight years old and living a life that was definitely 'on hold' until I could retire. I was convinced that because I had adopted a particular kind of attitude, and practised a certain kind of approach to my life for the past twenty years, that I could continue repeating that approach for the next twenty years and it would not make a difference. I adopted the 'if it worked then, it will work now' attitude. Of course this was an illusion. Changing the way I saw things was essential if I wanted the free, enriched, wild, rare life past sixty that I rightfully deserved. I could not see a way out because I was attached to the ideas that I held about my working life, health, home and myself.

Creating The MACE Pathway helped me to bring movement, action, creativity, and enjoyment into my life because it is a process of aliveness and discovery. The MACE Pathway is a guide to living your life as the splendid, bold remarkable you. It is about remembering that we all are forgivable, loveable and creative colourful beings.

Introducing The MACE Pathway

Bring to mind a huge, beautiful and ancient mountain. This awesome mountain represents your life as it is right now. As you look up you may shrink and feel tiny, powerless and frustrated. The MACE Pathway supports us in considering the choices we are making in our lives. Sometimes the most alive choices feels like a bit of a risk, some can make us giggle and some can make the hairs on the back of our neck stand up. Some of our choices can be tiny, some can be large, some can be simple and some can be a completely new route. The MACE Pathway walks you around the mountain of your life, gradually ascending in a spiral. As the pathway ascends the mountain it gives its walker the opportunity to breathe, using all their senses to explore what they experience and to examine how they feel about the challenges in their life, posing questions about changing the way they see things now.

The mountain spiral pathway represents:

- The creation of something new through the harmony between mind and body.
- Endless lessons available to be learnt.
- Life as the unravelling of new ideas and opportunities.
- Life as full of hope, endless possibility, growth and vitality.
- The beauty of simplicity.

With The MACE Pathway, we do not ascend by going straight up. We would become exhausted, facing and stumbling over and around boulders and rivers in our path. The mountain spiral path of The MACE Pathway means that we walk gently around but still ascend the mountain, using all our senses to enjoy the moments, experiences, and explorations whilst unfurling life's possibilities.

I created The MACE Pathway because change happens. The one thing we can be certain of is that change will occur in our lives. No matter how much we fear it, it happens. We are living through times of great change that affects all areas of our life whether at home, work or at leisure. Change is affecting how our children learn. Times of change require choices to be made; some choices lead to action and some choices lead to inaction. Living through the turmoil of change can be unsettling. Either way there are consequences, and those consequences affect our lives. We forget that we are splendid, bold and remarkable, and sometimes during a time of difficult change we think that it would be easier to wait until the change passes, before continuing on with our dreams and the plans we have for our life.

The impact of change on my life was that I had totally put my life on hold, which was having disastrous effects. My mid-life had certainly given me one challenging journey to unravel and it had been triggered by losing sight of what was important to me. Each working day I seemed to magnetise stress towards myself. As the stress created more confusion and powerlessness I began to sink fast. I looked around me for support, either in the form of a book, a course, or a person. I was seeking anything that I could use to help me to make sense of my situation, and to empower me to see the positive side of being in my mid-life and heading towards retirement.

What made me change the way I saw things?

It was the day those 17 years flashed in bright neon colours in front of me. John, a perfect stranger who was selling insurance had said to me, 'Elaine, I have found that people tend to live until they are seventy-five-years-old, give or take a few years.' He then asked me the question that tipped my life headlong into a process of changing the way I saw things. 'How many years have you got left?' Only 17 pulsed brightly in front of me. I thought about it over and over and over again. 17 years. 17!

It was late 2010, I was fifty-eight years old and I was walking away from a teaching career of over thirty years. I loved teaching and I chose it as a career because I was passionate about making a difference. My schooling experience was unsuccessful and miserable. As a mature student living in the 1960s and 1970s UK, I was able to gain a degree, a teaching qualification and a Masters.

This experience gave me the passion, drive and enthusiasm to become a qualified teacher, and the determination to make a difference by providing education that supports and enhances belonging, identity and equality. My work as a teacher had always excited me and filled me with energy. But now I was living a life consumed by stress, fatigue and without direction.

I became interested in self-help and personal leadership in the early 1990s when my marriage broke up, and I became an unsupported single parent overnight. I read avidly, attempting to apply 'uplifting' techniques to my own life. The early work of

Virginia Satir (See bibliography) broke new ground for me and I attended a personal development training course called Outlook. This training enabled me to see my life from different points of view and gave me a tool kit to manage my life.

I had many conversations with my peers as I faced crises and challenges. As a fifty-eight year old woman, I felt my life was deteriorating fast. Some of my peers called what I was going through a 'mid-life crisis'. I was slowly realising that it was time to live the life I wanted to live, and not the life I thought I was supposed to. If I wanted to step out of my world of stress, fatigue, low self-esteem and powerlessness. I needed to embrace the rest of my life with movement, action, creativity and enjoyment and continue to make a difference. I had to change the way I saw things, now.

By late 2010, I was seriously closed down and unaware and I rarely socialised with family and friends. My reading, cinema and exhibition visits, which I used to love, had shrunk. All of life's small challenges became problems, which mushroomed out of control, overnight. This viewpoint led me to believe that I was trapped and powerless in my situation and with no escape. I believed that any decisions that I made would lead me directly into disaster and insecurity. My self-trust eroded daily. My fundamental belief was that I had no choice but to continue in my situation. I was a victim waiting for someone else to give me permission.

My life was out of balance. I was eating unhealthily with far too much carbohydrate and refined sugar in my diet. I drank tea and coffee rather than water. Exercise was something I read and talked about but rarely actually did. I used white wine to anesthetise me from my life and chocolate and chips to comfort me. From this closed-down, out-of-balance ungrounded place, I lived my life going around in ever decreasing circles. My sense of purpose was long gone and everything became a drag. I slipped lower and lower into a puddle of powerlessness.

Through my stressful working life I had gradually burnt myself out. My life was full of hassles, deadlines, frustrations, and demands. Stress was so commonplace that it had become a way of life. I understood that stress wasn't always bad, and in small doses it could help with performance, indeed, under pressure, stress can be a motivator. However the stress in my life had gone beyond a certain point and was not helpful. It began causing damage to my health, mood, focus, effectiveness, relationships and quality of life. Living a life submerged by stress I couldn't see that things could be different. During this time of challenge, I struggled and picked over and picked at my life. I squeezed, pushed and pulled at myself trying to ascertain why my life seemed to be empty of love, trust and belief in myself.

Our personal stories are powerful

As I wrote *The Time for Freedom* my story appeared on my laptop screen before me. It looked like an endless stream of stumblings, resistances, complaints, refusals, obsessions, and ravings. I also heard my inner voice continually saying 'no one will be interested in this! Who else feels this way? You are the only one who feels like this!' With this loud and negative self-talk, it was difficult not to believe that I was alone with my experiences. However as I gave my story airtime, and I spoke to people attending my workshops up and down the country and to colleagues, associates, neighbours and friends, I realised that what I had experienced during the years 2005 to 2010 was not unusual. Mine was a common story of the struggle between living the life I thought I should live and the one I wanted to live, and the stress and tension that is created through this internal and external struggle. For me it occurred in my late 50s. For some it was occurring in their 30s, others in their 40s, 60s, 70s, and 80s. We are never too young or old to be affected by these feelings.

Some of my story is dark, and when I read it I think I have written the unspeakable. I have expressed my 'stuck-ness', my repetition of negative patterns, my feeling of being lost. I have chosen to share my story and life experiences through my writing to provide evidence that none of us is alone in our feelings. The context of my personal story took place in a school in east London. However, my experience is played out in many of our lives, across the UK, Europe and the world. I have written about things that really happened to me, even when it was unflattering. I believe that when we share 'real stuff' we have the power to alchemise it into something valuable that we can bring into the world through creating community. I believe that we are so full of glorious treasures that the stories of our lives can create huge libraries containing gems and other treasures that become available to share with others.

Through introspection I created some clarity in my life

I sat down one chilly autumn day with a pot of tea and *The Bhagavad Gita*. The 'Gita' as it is referred to, is an ancient Sanskrit text and is a manual of action. It is about how to 'be' in the material life and at the same time how to be spiritual. It is a dialogue between a teacher who is Krishna and his pupil Arjuna that happened over 5,000 years ago Arjuna is a great warrior prince living in India. He is standing on a battlefield facing the greatest challenges of his life. As Arjuna questions, wonders and panics about the possible situations and failures he may face, he is challenged by Krishna. Krishna imparts learning, and this learning enables Arjuna to rise to the very pinnacle of his human potential and be victorious against impossible odds. Arjuna is all of us and his challenges are our lifetime challenges. His victory is ours. I use this book daily as it always has something new to share.

As I picked up my copy of *The Bhagavad Gita* on that autumn day, a piece of paper with the simple but very powerful Serenity Prayer written on it fell out:

Grant me the serenity to accept the things that cannot be changed,
the courage to change the things that I can,
and the wisdom to know the difference.

The Serenity Prayer motivated me to write in my journal. As I wrote, the pages in my journal began to fill with my words and interesting ideas began to take shape. Acceptance! Courage! Change! Wisdom! Difference! I gained clarity that I had lived the life I was 'supposed' to live. Now I should live the life I *wanted* to live. To enable me to make the right choices it was important for me to change the way I saw things. This was my call to action. As I wrote I evolved my mountain visualisation. Visualisation or guided imagery is a process that affects every aspect of your body. I sat with my back firmly against the chair and my feet flat on the floor. I was relaxed and focused on the pictures my mind was creating.

Mountain visualisation

In front of me was a beautiful and ancient mountain, which was huge.

I imagined myself taking steady steps along the path making a spiral ascent. In one pocket was a small flask of Chai. Chai is a mixture of black tea and spices and makes a comforting and warming drink.

I saw myself ascending the mountain. Not climbing straight up but taking the scenic, longer route. Walking around the mountain. Walking upwards in a spiral.

I was barefoot, and enjoying feeling Mother Earth beneath me.

I was mindful of every step I took. How and where I placed my foot.

As I walked I was also mindful of using all my senses to record my walk.

I considered which relationships, experiences, knowledge, skills and understanding had nurtured me. I gave love, gratitude, and acknowledgement to the important people in my life.

On arrival at the top of the mountain, I found a comfortable and safe place to sit. I poured a cup of Chai and reflected upon my collection of thoughts from my spiral ascent, while sipping my Chai. When I had completed and explored all my thoughts, experiences and feelings I tightened the lid to my flask and replaced the cup.

I stood up and took in a deep breath before beginning my descent. I was mindful as I walked of my adventure and open to the possibilities it had revealed.

Upon arrival at my starting point I felt the earth under my feet and the breeze on my face. Standing still like the mountain, open to what life may bring. I gently opened my eyes.

I used what I had gathered from my visualisation to consider my next steps. I wrote and drew in my journal, using many different coloured pens. Something interesting began to emerge and that was The MACE Pathway.

The MACE Pathway explained

The visualisation and my recordings in my journal allowed me to gently listen to my inner whispers and ideas. These guided me to gain clarity and create a structure and The MACE Pathway emerged. The mountain is a metaphor of our life and the upward spiral path is the path of ascent to our best life. The path does not go straight up but carefully and intently goes around the mountain, an opportunity to take in the view and explore ideas:

- The **M**ACE Pathway: **M**e.
- The M**A**CE Pathway: **A**ttitude.
- The MA**C**E Pathway: **C**ommitment.
- The MAC**E** Pathway: **E**njoyment.

Chapter 1. The <u>M</u>ACE Pathway: <u>ME</u>

The 'M' in Mace focuses my attention firmly on me. I understood that to change the way I saw things, it was important to become aware of how I was seeing things now. Before I could think of where I wanted to go to, or what outcome I wanted to create, I needed to know where I was. The MACE Pathway: ME includes my personal story and invites you to consider different strategies for exploring yourself through:

- Personal paradigms and, self-awareness
- I would rather be right than happy
- Stress and recognising its symptoms
- Limiting beliefs
- Affirmations
- Event plus response equals outcome
- Finding a sense of Purpose
- Making a Choice, and creating Freedom
- Conclusion
- Pathway Gems

Chapter 2. The M<u>A</u>CE Pathway: <u>A</u>TTITUDE

Focusing on the 'A' in MACE is about taking responsibility and making decisions about attitude choices. I felt powerless in my own life and experienced immobilisation. I wanted control over my own life, but I didn't have the self-belief to support me there. My continuous attitude of self-doubt plunged me deeper into 'I'm not good enough.' I have included my personal story information, insight, ideas and strategies about:

- Positive thinking
- Changing the way we see things gives our subconscious positive messages

- Perfectionism
- Comparison
- Blame
- Challenging my attitude
- Finding self-compassion
- From: Do Be Have to Be Do Have
- Conclusion.
- Pathway Gems

Chapter 3. The MACE Pathway: COMMITMENT

Commitment or a call to action is an acceptance of self-journey and exploration, but also a clear understanding of the role of commitment in creating change. In this part there is a clear direction towards the positive aspects of goal setting and getting. Once we set ourselves small goals and we attain them, we learn that we can make a difference to our lives. As we scale up those goals we ultimately realise that we are hugely powerful beings that can make an amazing difference to our own lives and the lives of people around us. I have included my personal story and information, insight, ideas and strategies about:

The MACE Pathway: COMMITMENT

- Dream dare do!
- Listen to your whispers
- What is commitment?
- Why set goals?
- A question of time
- Setting a goal is not about the future; it brings clarity here and now

- How does Positive thinking affect our goal getting?
- Conscious and subconscious mind
- Our thoughts affect our thinking
- Making that commitment to your goal
- Some reasons that can stop us from successful goal getting
- Goal Mapping
- Bringing my Goals Alive!
- Conclusion
- Pathway Gems

Chapter 4. The MAC<u>E</u> Pathway – <u>E</u>NJOYMENT!

The E in MACE focused me on enjoyment. Working a 12-hour day, I had so much to do and so little time, that the idea of spending time doing anything that was unrelated to my to do list completely stressed me out. I had convinced myself that anything that brought joy to my life was a waste of time. Having the 'E' in The MACE Pathway supported me to look closely at enjoyment and to claim it back. As well as my personal story, I have included the following:

The MACE Pathway: ENJOYMENT!

- Balance and Wellbeing
- Health
- Rest, relaxation and sleep for health
- Yoga
- Meditation
- Walking
- Celebrating personal stories

- Finding the beauty and truth in the ordinary
- Creating community
- Giving
- Conclusion
- Pathway Gems

Conclusion

Walking The MACE Pathway enabled me to change the way I saw things and I successfully transformed my life from one of stress and powerlessness into one of creating a new beginning and freedom. There were ups and there were downs but I learnt that the trick is to enjoy the ride.

A Story - Carrot, Egg, or Coffee Bean?

You will never look at a cup of coffee the same way again.

A young woman went to her mother and told her about her life and how things were so hard for her. She did not know how she was going to make it and wanted to give up. She was tired of fighting and struggling. It seemed that as one problem was solved, a new one arose.

Her mother took her to the kitchen. She filled three pots with water and placed each on a high heat. Soon the pots came to boil. In the first, she placed carrots, in the second she placed eggs, and the last she placed ground coffee beans. She sat and let them boil, without saying a word.

After about twenty minutes she turned off the burners. She fished out the carrots and placed them in a bowl. She pulled out the eggs and placed them in a bowl. Then the ladled the coffee out and placed it in the bowl.

Turning to her daughter she said, 'Tell me, what do you see?'

She brought her closer and asked her to feel the carrots. The daughter did and noted that they were soft. The mother then asked her to take an egg and break it. After pulling off the shell, her daughter observed the hard-boiled egg. Finally she asked her to sip the coffee. The daughter smiled, as she tasted its rich aroma.

The daughter then asked, 'What does all this mean, mother?'

Her mother explained that each of these objects had faced the same adversity – boiling water – but each had reacted differently. The carrots went in strong, hard and unrelenting. However, subjected to boiling water they softened and became weak. The egg had been fragile with its strong outer shell protecting its liquid interior but after sitting in boiling water it had become hardened. The ground coffee beans were unique, however. The boiling water hadn't changed them – they had changed the water.

'Which are you?' She asked her daughter. 'When adversity knocks on your door, how do you respond? Are you a carrot, an egg or a coffee bean?' Think of this: Which am I? Am I the carrot that seems strong, but weakens with pain and adversity? Do I wilt and become soft and lose my strength?'

Which are you?

Are you the egg that starts with a malleable heart, but changes with the heat? Did you have a fluid spirit, but after a death, a breakup, a financial hardship or some other trial, become hardened and stiff? Does your shell look the same, but on the inside you are bitter and tough with a stiff spirit and a hardened heart?

Or are you like the coffee bean? The bean actually changes the hot water – the very circumstance that brings the pain. When the water gets hot, it releases the fragrance and flavour of your life. If you are like the bean, when things are at their worst, you get better and change the situation around you. When the hours are the darkest and trials are their greatest, you elevate to another level.

How do you handle adversity? Are you changed by your surroundings or do you bring life, and flavour to them?

Are you a carrot, an egg or a coffee bean?

Author Unknown

By 2010, there is no doubt that I was living my life in adverse conditions. I believe that through doing what I thought I couldn't I have learnt an invaluable life-changing lesson. That is that anything is possible – in my life I did what scared me the most. I left my comfortable lifetime career of over thirty years and stepped out of my comfort zone and took early retirement. I committed to a new beginning and I created The MACE Pathway I listened to my whispers and held possibility close to my heart. So can you.

Pathway Gems

Captured Thoughts:

'The greatness of a man or woman is not in how much wealth he or she acquires, but in his or her integrity and his or her ability to affect those around him or her positively.'

Bob Marley, Singer/songwriter and musician

Movement, Action, Creativity and Enjoyment

Movement – Spinal Twist

Using activations to move our bodies is both nourishing and stimulating. It improves and regulates the energy flow within the whole body and prepares your body for movement. Activations warm our bodies up and prepare them for movement, start slowly and gradually build up the momentum, allowing your body to warm up at its own rhythm and pace. Repeat each exercise until you feel your body loosening.

Spinal Twist

Separate your feet to shoulder-width. Begin to twist your body to the right and then to the left. Lead the twist with your hips, allowing your body and arms to follow. Let your arms swing loosely so that they wrap around your body at the end of each twist. Turn your head in the direction of the twist and allow your arms to swing up higher with each twist. To increase the twist you can come onto the ball of your left foot as you twist to the right and onto the ball of your right foot as you twist to the left.

Action – Morning Pages

Julia Cameron's concept of Morning Pages comprise three pages of longhand writing. A consciousness stream. An end-less stream of whatever is in your mind or heart. There is no judgment when writing your Morning Pages, so there are no good, bad, wrong or right Morning Pages. For Julia Cameron, 'Pages' are meant to be, simply, the act of moving the hand across the page and writing down whatever comes to mind.' When writing my own Morning Pages nothing is too small, too big, too weird, too stupid or too clever to write about. Any-thing and everything can be included if I want it to be.

Action – Rise and Shine

When you wake up in the morning, completely relax your body for one minute, while you're still lying in bed. Think of five things you're really grateful for. Then gently sit up and wrap your duvet around you. Bring your attention to your breathing and let it get deeper without forcing it at all. Focus on your heart and feel warmth spreading through your body as you breathe. Continue for five minutes, then stretch and start your day.

Creativity – capturing your whispers

I invite you to use all or some of these prompts and record your responses in whatever creative way you choose.

- In the depths of my heart, creative dreams are calling me to take notice. They are:
- The one thing I never thought I could do is:
- Here's how I can do it:
- Who in my life has passion? What questions could I ask him/her? What is their story?

- I feel most inspired when:

Enjoyment is about having fun along the way. Not worrying about what others may think, feel, say or do. It is about your nourishment. Do what you need to do today to bring Enjoyment into your life.

Chapter 1

THE MACE PATHWAY: ME

In 2010 I realised that changing the way I saw things now began with focusing on myself. During the latter part of my teaching career I would start projects and not follow them through. I would agree to do things that I did not want to do simply because I thought I should. I sought comfort by consuming unhelpful food and drink, for example refined sugar and alcohol. I didn't enjoy what I watched on TV. I used up copious amounts of energy persuading others to do things for me. I began to fall asleep during meetings, on the bus and in the car. My life, which included my career path, was failing me. I felt like a beached whale! It was clear that I had reached a time in my life when changing the way I saw things needed to happen immediately and the process began with me.

As with any journey that required directions, to guide me I also required an identified starting point. For example, if I wanted to drive to Southend-on-Sea in Essex and I had no idea where it was, I would use a map to find its location and also to guide me there. If I was travelling from Bournemouth, I would take one route, from Colchester another and from Bangor another. Knowing where I was and where I wanted to get to was essential planning for clarity on any journey and this self-journey in particular However, if I were unable to identify where I was, a map, no matter how detailed, would offer no direction at all. I needed to sort out where I was and what I wanted.

Personal paradigms and self-awareness.

I have been inspired by the work of Brian Mayne and in particular something I read in *Goal Mapping The Practical Workbook* He states that 'A paradigm is a general viewpoint that we hold about something or someone and acts as a guidance grid for our opinions, attitudes and actions. Each paradigm that we hold is like a personal picture of understanding that we project onto the world and everything in it. It is the map or blueprint that our subconscious constantly reads to regulate our actions and reactions.'

Our personal pictures or paradigms work for us, because it means that we do not need to be constantly working out who we are and how we need to deal with our world. We build up personal paradigm pictures of ourselves acting and reacting in lots of different ways across different situations in our lives. Our personal pictures of ourselves work for us when we want to carry out tasks that are routine, for example, drive a car, cycle to the shops, walk to the park. These activities that many of us take for granted are achieved without conscious effort because it is our subconscious that is carrying them out.

Personal paradigms do work for us for most of our lives. However, there is a challenge in that once we create a paradigm we can make it in concrete and we can fix it solidly. And we may then become unwilling to change it.

I had reached mid-life and I did not understand why my life was deteriorating. For over fifty years the world of work had been in my consciousness, and it had ploughed a deep groove through my life. It began with childhood questions about what I wanted to do when I grew up, then later, at school the questions were around examination choices. Later still they became questions on which area of work I was going to apply for. My choices of work were limited and narrow and mainly revolved around typing and shorthand so I was dissatisfied with my options. Then came the 1970s when a strong societal belief evolved that anything and everything was possible. I enrolled in night school and passed GCE O Level and A Level exams, enabling me to enrol on a degree course. Having BA after my name meant I could participate in a different world of work, and I successfully became a teacher.

Over time, one thing I did discover about life was that change happens. However, I feared it. For example, in the 21st Century change is fast and furious and the careers that today's pre-school children will follow have not yet been invented.

Back then, I had a very clear personal paradigm about retirement. When I thought about it a multitude of negative, uninspiring, unempowering, and unhelpful images of women of 60-plus years of age came into my mind. I conjured up pictures of old age that involved blue rinses, cruises, loss of energy, illness, loss of interest and boredom. Fear of old age is not a new concept. As I got older, sometimes I referred to myself as 'being old' instead of expressing gratitude for having reached an age of wisdom and understanding. I certainly felt that once over 60, no one would listen to my ideas or take me seriously ever again.

Then, along with retirement, came the grief attached to the loss of my contribution to society and self-respect through the loss of my identity. I had completely lost sight of positive role models such as the brilliant actress Sheila Hancock, the amazing author and leader Germaine Greer, and the incredible author and editor Diana Athill. I had also overlooked a 'posse' of dynamic, inspiring, adventurous family and friends who were aged 60+ who acted as role models in my life.

This turmoil led to unhappiness with my life and I was finding it difficult to consider my options. I could be dead in 17 years so did I have time to waste? I lived in a constant fog of being unaware of the outcomes of my actions and of my inactions. I was blundering around in my life. I had a limited viewpoint, which was that I had to stay at my place of work for the next four years and there was no way out. This was a distorted paradigm that I was attached to and I was unaware at the time that it was leading me into a narrow and closed attitude and an uncreative outlook. This was digging a big hole in which I was burying all my dreams and passions. I was behaving as a victim, and I had lost all sense that this lifestyle was my choice.

I would rather be right than happy

I began to look at, and to challenge my personal viewpoints of my life. At various points during my life I had turned my opinions, attitudes, behaviour and my outcomes, into truths. And believing that they were truths, I had made them 'right' and protected them. One truth I had protected and made right, was that even though it was very stressful and making me very miserable, there was only one way to manage my working life, and that was to stay in full time teaching until I became of pensionable age. As someone once said, 'I would rather be right than happy.' And they were right!

My paradigm shift that began with the question from John had motivated me to create action and energy to craft a new beginning for myself. I was taking the baby steps of a major life change. As in life, baby steps invariably contain obstacles, slopes to clamber up, hurdles to climb over, steep slopes to get down and ruts that involve problem-solving to get out of. I remember watching Max my son, tackle the process of learning to walk. He had a positive outlook and he approached this process full of curiosity and excitement. When we think positively, chemicals that are released in our brains generate brain-cell connections, which help us produce new ideas, answers and solve problems. Negative thoughts block creativity and cause negative thoughts to be formed. While learning to walk Max invariably fell down or his experiment didn't work out. He didn't blame me, the furniture or anyone else in the room. Because of his positive attitude he gave a little chuckle and carried on taking the risks, making the mistakes and enjoying the process, which eventually led to his success as a walking toddler. When I reflected on Max's learning to walk process, I could see how I could apply it to my life in my present situation.

Having a positive attitude and venturing to do something new, being willing to take risks and not giving up on myself while I made mistakes, was a good starting point from which to approach my situation in 2010. I also needed to hear and see the feedback I was receiving about my attitude, learn from it and use it creatively as a motivator to take action. Taking these small but powerful baby steps supported me to the next phase of my life.

Stress and recognizing its symptoms

Being alive means experiencing stress. Stress as a positive influence helps us move forward, helps us get into action. With this kind of stress we achieve and succeed. On the other hand, stress as a negative influence leads to numerous health problems. Stress makes us fearful and angry and can lead to depression. Stress speeds aging and can kill us, swiftly and without warning. Or slowly because our lives have been out of balance for a long time.

Unhealthy stress happens because we have too much to do, because we feel we are not in control and because change is happening too fast. Stress has become our constant companion because our lives have become too complicated. We have forgotten the beautiful moments of simplicity. We think that this is just the way it is. The world is moving at a frantic pace and we move anxiously with it.

Reducing and managing stress is about establishing a point of balance in our lives. It is about learning how to get off the roller coaster, how to think less and literally how to be more in the here and now. When we learn how to do this, we realise that the here and now is about a series of single moments that can be experienced without the stressors we have become so used to.

Sometimes we do not recognise that we are stressed because we slowly adapt to the increasing pressures that we experience and we come to accept them as 'normal.' We usually experience stress when our resources are not sufficient to cope with the pressures and demands from the environment. But stress can also be caused by too little stimulation. A certain amount of stimulation is necessary for us to be motivated and to perform well, we just need to achieve the right balance for us so that we can achieve the optimum outcomes without compromising our well-being.

We experience burn out and ill health when we push ourselves beyond fatigue for too long, whereas low levels of arousal for anything but a short time can lead to boredom, lethargy and depression. Everyone has their own unique stress curve; some people have a much higher tolerance for stress and need stimulation, whilst others tolerate stress poorly.

Stress has more to do with ourselves and with our perception and reaction to situations, than it has with the situation itself. For one person an exam or test may be stressful, but someone else may experience it as a challenge and an opportunity. Some of us would be terrified at the thought of bungee jumping, whilst others do this for fun. The lesson is that if we know ourselves better and keep ourselves balanced, then the world is more likely to be experienced in a positive way and we are less likely to experience events as stressful.

Limiting beliefs

My beliefs about myself were limiting me. I had limiting beliefs about my success, my capabilities and how I related to people. The day I realised that I had these negative beliefs about myself was the day I took my first step towards doing and creating something different.

Through my journal writings, I was able to see that I had set myself short-, medium- and long-term goals, however I had not accomplished any of them. I had built within myself a strong limiting belief that I was not capable of accomplishing anything that I wanted to achieve. I told myself that 'I can't do that; I don't know how to do that; I'm too old.' And the one limiting belief that had really stood in my way for quite a few years: 'my writing is not good enough to be published'. Deep inside I wanted to write and publish a book that would make a difference to its readers by changing the way they saw things. Instead of the negative story that I repeatedly told myself, I wanted to give myself different beliefs, 'I can do this; I am capable; If I do need support with my writing, there is someone out there who can support and teach me.' I began to look at strategies for making a shift to seeing myself as competent, which would mean that I began to see my life differently. Instead of living in the past and thinking about what I could have had, I was now thinking in the present about what I wanted to accomplish in my life. The difference was enormous, and top of my list of what I wanted to accomplish in my life was the publication of a book, which of course, is *The Time for Freedom*.

I also had another internal dialogue. I didn't believe that I was competent enough to handle my life's challenges. My limiting beliefs were undermining my self-esteem. Then, one day I was reflecting and looking through my archived journals and I could clearly see, from what I had written that I had handled challenging situations in my life. I left home when I was quite young; I looked after and cared for myself; I managed when my mum became ill; I coped when my dad died; when my marriage fell apart; when I had to have my cat put to sleep. All those things were tough but I handled them. I am sure you have handled difficult situations too and you can handle anything else that happens to you as well. Once I understood that, my confidence began to grow. I began to believe in myself and know that I was capable of handling anything that came up in my life.

When I talk to people in my workshops about limiting beliefs, in addition to believing that they are incapable, or somehow not deserving of acknowledgment they add limiting beliefs of their own such as:

- I'm not young enough.
- I don't look like that.
- Women don't do that sort of thing.
- I'd never make head teacher.
- I'm not smart enough.
- Nothing I do works.

The process I use when limiting beliefs creep into my thoughts is detailed within the Action in the following Pathway Gens,.

Affirmations

Affirmations are positive statements that describe a desired situation, and which are repeated many times, in order to impress the subconscious mind and trigger it into positive action. In order to ensure the effectiveness of the affirmations, they have to be repeated with attention, conviction, interest, and desire.

Imagine that you are walking with your friends. They are going to walk up the local high mountain. Something you have never done before. You start walking and at the same time keep repeating in your mind, I can do it, I can do it. You keep thinking and believing that you are going to get to the top. What you are actually doing is repeating positive affirmations.

Many of us repeat in our minds negative words and statements concerning the situations and events in our lives, and consequently, create undesirable situations. Words and statements work both ways, to build or destroy. It is the way we use them that determines whether they are going to bring good or harmful results. Sometimes we repeat negative statements in our mind, without even being aware of what we are doing. Actually, we are sending a message to our subconscious mind that it accepts as true. When we say to ourselves; I am lazy, or I am stupid, or I am bad. Etc., Our subconscious mind believes these statements and eventually attracts corresponding events and situations into our lives; irrespective whether they are good or bad for us.

Affirmations program the mind in the same way that commands and scripts program a computer. The repeated words help us to focus our mind on our aim, and automatically build corresponding mental images in the conscious mind, which affect the subconscious mind, in a similar manner. The conscious mind, the mind you think with, starts this process, and then the subconscious mind takes charge. By using this process consciously and intently, you can affect your subconscious mind, and thereby, transform your habits, behaviour, mental attitude, and reactions, and even reshape your external life. Sometimes, results appear quickly, but often more time is required. Depending on your goal, sometimes, you might attain immediate results, and at other times, it might take days, weeks, months or more. Getting results depends on several factors, such as the time, focus, faith and feelings you invest in repeating your affirmations, on the strength of your desire, and on how big or small is your goal. It is important to understand that repeating positive affirmations for a few minutes, and then thinking negatively the rest of the day, neutralizes the effects of the positive words. You have to refuse to think negative thoughts, if you wish to attain positive results.

Event plus response equals outcome

I attended a Jack Canfield course held in Santa Barbara, USA, a few years ago. He taught and demonstrated this simple but valuable formula that helped make the idea of 100 per cent responsibility clear to me.

$$\text{Event} + \text{Response} = \text{Outcome}$$

Or

$$E+R=O$$

All outcomes in our lives are the result of how we have responded to an earlier event or events in our lives. Those outcomes can relate to health or illness, intimacy or estrangement, joy or frustration, success or failure, wealth or poverty.

The formula can be explained in the following way.

If I do not like the outcome that I am getting, I have two choices that I can make:

1. I could blame the event (E) for my unhappy outcome (O)

or

2. I could change my response (R) to the event (E) until I get the outcome (O) that I want.

From 2005 to 2010, I was blaming the event (E) for my lack of results. I blamed my working life for the powerless and dull life that I was living and I stopped myself progressing by not leaving. I believed in a number of excuses as to why I should put my life on hold and remain in my work, no matter what the situation was doing to me.

In 2010 I changed my response (R) to the events (E) and I slowly but surely began to get the outcomes (O) that I wanted. I changed the way I saw things and I decided to do, think and say things differently. I questioned my communication, I changed my images of myself and my work and I changed my behaviour. I claimed back my power and changed the way I interacted with the world. I felt like a bundle of reflexes and I wanted to regain control of my thoughts, dreams, daydreams and my behaviour. I wanted intention to be at the root of everything I thought, said, and did.

Many people overcome limiting factors in their lives. It seems to me that we regularly think limiting thoughts and engage in self-defeating behaviours. There were times when I even defended my self-destructive habits, for example alcohol abuse, with quite indefensible logic. In the years leading up to 2010 I was firmly placing the blame for everything that wasn't the way I wanted it on circumstances. I had an excuse for everything. But I learnt that we have the freedom to respond how we choose to respond in any given situation. Taking that responsibility can:

- Inspire our minds.

- Motivate our emotions.

- Bring purpose to our behaviour.
- Empower our habits.

This is taking responsibility. By choosing to take responsibility, you put yourself in the driving seat of your life where feedback and learning is your guide, and you can live a life of freedom.

Finding a sense of Purpose

We are not all motivated by the same things. I was an enthusiastic and dedicated teacher who was passionate about the rights of children. I was and am serious about making a difference, and for much of my life, my work and my purpose was in alignment. I strove to be a good teacher, always going the extra mile and keeping up to date with current ideas and trends. I was passionate about creating learning environments that worked for everyone, with no one left out.

Through my lifetime of experiences and wisdom, I became clear about my purpose. Being in alignment with my Life Purpose has supported and motivated me. It has helped me see that it is important for me to do what I love to do, and to accomplish what is important to me.

My Life Purpose is: To inspire and empower children, women and men to love, trust and believe in themselves, changing the way they see things now, so they can live a great life.

Here are some Life Purpose statements of some friends of mine:

- Inspire the world to create peace in a heartbeat.
- Create a world where the sun shines continuously in every person's heart.
- Create a world that works for everyone with no one left out.

I believe that each of us is born with a Life Purpose. Identifying, acknowledging and honouring this purpose can be the most important action that we take. Being clear about your Life Purpose will ensure that you are guided towards setting goals and action plans that evolve into success. I would like to support you in unearthing your Life Purpose. In the Action section of Pathway Gems there is an exercise you can work through to support you in becoming clear about your Life Purpose.

Making a choice, and creating Freedom

The Time For Freedom could be considered by some as a 'grand' title; it is certainly ambitious. Knowing that I can choose my response is actually my greatest freedom. I am constantly humbled by the ordinary children, women and men who in their daily lives courageously speak their truth, stand up for what is important to them and show up for who they are. Their struggles have challenged the way we live our lives and have moulded our world today.

All things are created by a thought. Someone had an idea and at some point that thought was manifested. A thought led to Mary Seacole challenging what was expected of her, Van Gogh painting Sunflowers, Mansukh Patel creating the World Peace Flame, Sylvia Pankhurst setting up the East London Federation of Suffragettes, Bob Marley uniting the two sides of Jamaican politics in the 1970s, and Nelson Mandela having a pivotal role in ending Apartheid. The list is endless. All action and inaction begins with a thought. Everything that has ever been began with a thought.

In our lives our thoughts shape our world. I believed that I needed to tolerate my life and how I was living it and that I could do nothing about it. On a bad day, I could have described my weaknesses and given pages of reasons why I could not change or improve my life. I began to realise that all my reasons only told about what was influencing my life. I slowly began to see that although affecting my life, these reasons were not determining my life. I had the freedom to choose to improve my mental and emotional response, my outlook and my attitude. Slowly but surely what I unearthed was an understanding that I could choose to be the best I could be. I only need to change a thought. My freedom was beginning to be unearthed.

Conclusion

I was looking at myself, putting myself under a microscope and focusing on me, which made me feel uncomfortable and vulnerable. Vulnerability is owning what you have to own, wherever you may be in your life journey. This could be joy, confusion, gratitude happiness, and/or sadness. In my case, it was about nurturing and expressing something that needed attention in my life. At this point in my life I needed to pay attention, and honour all that was good in my life. At the same time I needed to nurture the part of me that was going to have to detach from the 'Elaine Mace Teacher' label. Embracing my vulnerability was about being honest with myself, honouring the truth that was inside me and saying what I really wanted for my life. Expression of my truth was at heart of The MACE Pathway: ME.

Pathway Gems

Captured Thoughts:

'When you are inspired by some great purpose, some extraordinary project, all your thoughts break their bonds; your mind transcends limitations, your consciousness expands in every direction and you find yourself in a new, great and wonderful world. Dormant forces, faculties and talents become alive and you discover you are a greater person by far than you ever dreamed yourself to be.'

Patanjali in *The Yoga Sutras*

'By being yourself you put something wonderful in the world that was not there before'

Sprinkle Joy Daily (sprinklejoy.com)

Movement, Action, Creativity and Enjoyment

Movement – The mountain posture

A mountain represents stability, strength and permanence. This very important posture can create stability and balance within us too. This is also the posture from which all yoga standing postures and sequences originate. It is important to stand in the posture with awareness and to focus on the various parts of yourself with the intention of bringing them into balance.

The mountain posture is the blueprint for all standing and movement postures in Dru Yoga. It awakens within you a feeling of strength and stability so that you can stand with confidence in your own power – just like a mountain. Awakening your inner strength and stability.

In the stillness that arises from physical and emotional alignment you can also experience a sense of unity between yourself and the world around you.

- Stand tall with your feet about hip-width apart (two fists wide) and your weight evenly distributed over the feet.

- Soften your knees slightly, checking that they are in line with your feet.

- Allow your arms to rest by your sides and your shoulders to relax.

- Gently lift the lower abdomen upwards and in to activate the core stability muscles.

- Lift from the sternum.

- Pull back slightly to help elongate the neck.

- Now imagine that the crown of your head is attached to a thread connected to the ceiling.

- Feel as it is softly pulling you upwards, elongating the whole of the spine.

- As you breathe in, feel the spine lengthen. As you breath out, feel the spine relax naturally back down.

- Now feel that you are breathing in through the crown of the head into your heart, and breathing out from your heart, down to your feet and into the earth.

- Feel that you are breathing in from the earth, back up to your heart and breathing out through your crown.

- Continue to breathe in this way until you feel a cantered connection with the world around you.

Silently affirm: I am a mountain of strength.

Action – A Stress-Busting Meditation

- Take the telephone off the hook and switch off any mobile phones.

- Go into a room, alone, where a calm and quiet atmosphere can be created, for approximately 20 minutes.

- Sit on a straight-backed chair or on the floor. It is important to sit alert and comfortable.

- Relax for a few moments and focus on breathing in and t.

- Pay attention to the natural rhythm of each inhalation and exhalation.

- Bring to mind a situation that brought you stress during the day. See the people. Get in touch with how you felt.

- Create an image of that situation in front of you, as if it were on a video screen.

- Breathe in through your nose, drawing some of the stress of the situation into your heart.

- Breathe out through your nose and visualise sending the stress out into the air so that it breaks up and blows away.

- Continue breathing the stress from the situation into your heart and then breathing it out, so that it blows away, until you see the situation as being completely healed.

- On an in-breath, draw this newly healed situation into your heart and breathe it out into the scene in front of you, bringing peace and a good solution to that situation. See smiles of relief on the faces of everyone concerned.

If you are experiencing stress from more than one situation, then repeat the above Action.

Action – Affirmations

Affirmations should be short and easy to remember and it is advisable to repeat them every time your mind is not engaged in something important, such as while traveling in a bus or a train, waiting in line, walking, etc., but do not affirm while driving or crossing a street. You may also repeat them in special sessions of 5-10 minutes each, several times a day. Examples of affirmations would be:

- I am healthy and happy.
- I am abundant.
- My mind is calm..
- I am surrounded by love.
- I have the perfect job for me.
- I am living in the house of my dreams.
- I have good and loving relations with my wife/husband.
- I am successful in whatever I do.

The Practice of Affirmations.

1. Close your eyes and relax any physical, emotional or mental tension while affirming. The stronger the concentration, the more faith you have in what you are doing, the more feelings you put into the act, the stronger and faster will be the results.

2. Decide on your affirmation. Choose only positive words, describing what you really want. If you desire to lose weight, do not tell yourself "I am not fat" or "I am losing weight." These are negative statements, bringing into the mind mental images of what you do not want. Say instead, "I am getting slim" or "I have reached my right weight". Such words evoke positive images in the mind.

51

3. Always affirm in the present tense, not the future tense. Saying, "I will be rich", means that you intend to be rich one day, in the indefinite future, but not now. It is more effective to say, and also feel, "I am rich now", and the subconscious mind will work at overtime to make this happen now, in the present.

The power of affirmations can help you to transform your life. By stating what you want to be true in your life, you mentally and emotionally see and feel it as true, irrespective of your current circumstances, and thereby attract it into your life.

Action – Squashing your Limiting Beliefs

This practical activity will support you to view and squash your limiting beliefs. Please work through the five points below:

1. Identify a limiting belief that you have of yourself that you would like to change. An example of some common limiting beliefs are: I'm stupid, I can't do anything right. I should hide what is really going on for me. It's not OK for me to share my feelings. What I think is not important.

2. Write it down.

3. With your limiting belief in front of you, determine and write down how that belief limits you.

4. Write down how you want to be, act, or feel.

5. Try to imagine how you could you turn your limiting belief into a positive belief, so that it gives you permission to be, act or feel in a new way.

Action – What is Your Purpose? Part One

I have used Robert Allen's four-quadrant method in my workshops with good results. Robert Allen is the co-author of The One Minute Millionaire. Allen classified the four quadrants into Talents, Passion, Values, and Intuition.

Talents are defined by what you are good at doing. Write down what you think you are good at. You can also talk about what you have written down with your friends and family members. Identify at least seven possible talents that you have. After that prioritise that top three and record them in the table below.

Passions can be defined by the things that you absolutely love to do. In your search for your purpose and meaning of life, you need to ask yourself seriously what the things that you would love to do are. These are usually things that you would do with energy and happiness. Once again, think of at least seven passions, and order the top three in the table.

Values can be defined as the things that you feel are the right things to do. In identifying the seven values items, it would help if you imagine that you only have five more years to live. Ask yourself what are the things that you absolutely must accomplish before you die.

The final quadrant is the Intuition quadrant. With this internal work we must not discount the hunches we have internally. Besides the analytical and mental approach to decision making, we have to depend on our sixth sense as well. Sometimes, all logical thinking might point towards a certain direction but your intuitive guidance says otherwise. Tap into this inner communication channel and identify seven things based on intuition. Select the top three and record them in the table below.

It is a good idea to complete the exercise to unearth your personal qualities. Find a quiet space that you know you will be undisturbed for about an hour. The key to this exercise is to idea is to find the common ground between each of these qualities.

Talents – what are three things I am really good at?	Passions – what are the three things that I absolutely love to do?
1 e.g. making cakes.	1 e.g. dance in the rain.
2	2
3	3
Values – what are the three things that it is essential that I must do, if I had five years left to live?	Intuition – what are the three things that I have a hunch that I should be doing?
1 e.g. walk daily no matter what the weather.	1 e.g. watercolour painting.
2	2
3	3

Once you have filled up all four quadrants in this exercise, look for any similar elements. Focus on the top three items in each quadrant. You will be able to identify one or two areas that appear in up to three quadrants. If you do have an item or two that appears in all four quadrants, than that's great. Start working on these.

Action – What is Your Purpose? Part Two

Using what you have unearthed using the quadrants.

1. Your personal qualities & characteristics

   Looking and using what you have unearthed using the quadrants, what do you think are your personal qualities. For example problem-solving, creativity, enthusiasm, ability to inspire, good leadership, compassionate, integrity, honesty, resourcefulness, and flexibility. Write down two of your strongest qualities. Qualities are not what you are good at doing they are what is important to you; what you hold dearly.

2. How do you enjoy or express those qualities in your life?

For each of these two qualities, write down how you enjoy expressing these in the things you do, say or think. Let's say you think you have a creative personality, perhaps you best enjoy expressing this quality by thinking of ideas for people to implement. You might also like to write novels or short stories that tell tales of the future in your free time. The way you express your personality has good implications about what life means to you.

3. A perfect world right now

Spend some time thinking about how this perfect world would look. Imagine all the vivid details in this world of yours. Who are the people you see and meet? How do they interact with each other? What are the trends of this world? How happy are the people? How does the world look physically? Let your imagination run wild.

4. Unearthing your purpose final steps

Write down a paragraph or two that combines all of the information that you have created. Be inclusive in this step. Write down as much detail as possible.

Action – What is Your Purpose? Part Three

When you feel that you have unearthed your purpose read it aloud. If you have goose bumps and can feel tears in your eyes, then you have touched your unique Life Purpose.

Record your Life Purpose both in writing and visually. Use colours to represent it. You may want to create a picture or symbol that represents your Life Purpose. Put it up on a wall or fridge; somewhere where it is visible to you regularly. This will help to keep you focused on what is important to you.

Here is what a workshop participant unearthed:

1. I am an adventurous and energetic speaker.

2. For adventure, I like to think of new ideas and implement them in all areas of my life. My friends and colleagues like to listen to me speak whenever there is a chance. They find my style engaging and energetic.

3. My perfect world is a peaceful place where people are all out to help each other to lead more empowered lives.

4. My purpose and meaning in life is to generate and implement new ideas to make the world a better place. I am destined to use my gifts of presentation to inspire people with these ideas for implementation.

Find a time and place to write where you won't be disturbed. Ideally, pick a time at the end of your workday or before you go to bed. Promise yourself that you will write for a minimum of 15 minutes a day, write continuously, and do not worry about spelling or grammar. Don't censor what you write. Write just for yourself. Some prompts to get you started could be your responses to the 'capturing your whispers' action.

Creativity – capture your whispers.

I invite you to use some or all of these prompts and record your thoughts in whatever creative way that you choose:

- The last time that I felt free spirited was:
- When it comes to my life, these are the fears I most need to recognise so I can move past them:
- If I wasn't afraid, I would:

- Write a list of the things that bring you happiness and joy. These can be from any aspect of your life.

- Write a separate list of the times that you have felt most happy, vibrant, and alive.

When it comes to embracing my hopes and passions, I can start with these small steps.

Enjoyment is about having fun along the way. Not worrying about what others may think, feel, say or do. It is about your nourishment. Do what you need to do today to bring Enjoyment into your life.

Chapter 2

THE MACE PATHWAY: ATTITUDE

I was clear that changing the way I saw things now was the way forward and the top of my agenda. I knew the MACE Pathway: ATTITUDE, would give me the structure, techniques and strategies that I needed to examine my unhelpful attitudes.

John's question challenged me, like a gauntlet thrown to the ground. My initial response was defence and confusion. However, underneath the pivotal question lay truths that needed my attention. I had calculated a possible 17 years of life. Did I want to waste my precious time feeling powerless, being stressed and being unhappy? The more I thought about this the more it sank deeper and deeper inside me and I unearthed the following attitudes:

- I had adopted a Peter Pan attitude that I thought I was going to live forever.

- I needed to accept that life was taking me closer towards old age.

- I had put off until tomorrow, things that could be organised today.

- My lack of work and life balance could be damaging my health.

John's poignant question made me focus on my attitudes and enabled me to see, focus on and accept some sharp home truths. The main one being that there was a chance that in 17 years times my body would not be so effective and I would be finding it difficult to live life to the full. It was time to get myself in order and pay attention to my attitudes. I was clear that I didn't just want to live my life – I wanted to live the width and depth of it.

The thought of wasting the next 17 years made me feel that I was letting myself down. I wanted to examine the attitudes that had brought me to this place, to consider a positive way forward and share what I had learnt.

Positive thinking

Positive thinking is a phrase that I have heard many times. It is so much a part of our vocabulary now that it has almost become meaningless. Positive thinking does not mean that you keep your head in the clouds and ignore life's less pleasant situations. Positive thinking just means that you approach the unpleasantness in a more positive, effective and productive way. You think the best is going to happen rather than the worst. Positive thinking often starts with self-talk. Self-talk is the endless stream of unspoken thoughts that run through our heads every day. These automatic thoughts can be positive or negative. Some of your self-talk comes from logic and reason; other self-talk may arise from misconceptions that you create because of lack of information. Much self-talk originates with our parents and sticks in our brains, replaying over and over again. If the thoughts that run through your head are mostly negative, your outlook on life is more likely pessimistic. If your thoughts are mostly positive, you're likely an optimist, someone who practises positive thinking. I've been honoured to meet people who remain happy most of the time and even during really challenging times. Over the past few years I have learnt much from them with regards to stillness, mindfulness, yoga and meditation.

Recently I have been reading about how positive thinking really does change thought patterns, in a real and physical way. The science that underpins this is called neuroplasticity. It means that our thoughts can change the structure and function of our brains. William James first introduced the idea in 1890, but scientists who uniformly believed the brain is rigidly mapped out, with certain parts of the brain controlling certain functions soundly rejected it.

They believed that if a part of the brain is dead or damaged, then the associated function is altered or lost. However it appears that they were wrong. Neuroplasticity now enjoys wide acceptance as scientist continue to prove that the brain is endlessly adaptable and dynamic. This means that repetitive positive thought and positive activity can rewire your brain and strengthen brain areas that stimulate positive feelings. The brain has the capacity to rewire itself and form new neural pathways but we need to work at it. Just like physical exercise, the work requires repetition and activity to reinforce new learning. The benefits positive thinking provide include:

- Increased life span.
- Lower rates of depression.
- Lower levels of distress.
- Greater resistance to the common cold.
- Better psychological and physical wellbeing.
- Reduced risk of death from cardiovascular disease.
- Better coping skills during hardship and times of stress.

It's unclear why people who engage in positive thinking experience these health benefits. One theory is that having a positive outlook enables us to cope better with stressful situations, which reduces the harmful health effects of stress on our bodies.

Changing the way we see things gives our subconscious positive messages

Our thoughts send messages to our amazing subconscious. It is widely known that we have two parts to our mind, one is our conscious mind and the other is our subconscious mind. Our conscious mind is our thinking mind, and is what is working right now to support you in reading this. Your subconscious is quite incredible, and works like a genie to your conscious mind. All your thoughts act as commands to your genie, your subconscious. Today we know that our conscious mind has huge power and works twenty-four hours a day. It is because of our subconscious that our body knows what to do while we are asleep. It manages habits, things we have learnt and behaviours. However scientists and doctors are still unsure about the overall capability of our subconscious mind.

I have learnt that with a change of attitude we can turn our possibilities into probabilities and our problems into challenges. Whether it is possibilities or probabilities or problems or challenges, depends on how we use our minds. No matter what is physically being demanded from us at the time. We are always free and able to choose our thoughts.

When I was attending primary and secondary school in the 1950s and 1960s I was firmly told by parents, family, teachers and people that cared for me and loved me that when I left school I would work in a office. During my working life, I would get married and have a family. I was told this many times and therefore I did believe that was my destiny. I did not believe there was any other option open to me. This belief lowered my expectations of myself and limited my outlook. A friend happened to ask if I had considered attending University. I came back with my answer in a moment 'Don't be ridiculous!'

However, that conversation sowed a seed that eventually led to me successfully completing a degree course and then a postgraduate certificate in education and a Masters. Nothing changed in my physical circumstances, I just chose to see things differently. Because of this change in attitude significant aspects of my life changed. It all began with a thought!

Perfectionism

I had always adopted the attitude towards work of giving 100 per cent, 100 per cent of the time. I always gave my work my best. When I began teaching, an elderly mentor gave me a tip. He told me that at the end of each day, I should reflect on the day. That I should write at the top of the day's space in my diary: 'how could I have improved that day?' I continued to do this throughout my career but by 2011 when I left teaching, my note in my diary was now headed 'what will they think?' I did not realise it, but living under the pressure of day-to-day stress, I had shifted my attitude from wanting to improve, to one of creating perfection. From reading books and discussing ideas with friends, family and colleagues, I became clear that there is a difference between perfectionism and being your best. I did not want to be perfect; however, perfectionism was something that had crept up on me, over a couple of years prior to 2010. I wanted to be perfect, because if I acted perfectly then I would minimise or even avoid colleague's judgements, blame, and even gossip.

My thoughts around perfectionism began to run all over my life. I had a deep fear of failing, and an even bigger fear of making mistakes and disappointing others. I could not take a risk. This was the opposite of what I wanted to create in the world. My ethos was; to learn you needed to take a risk, make a mistake and learning would take place. We like mistakes. I wanted to learn to love my mistakes again and to find some self-compassion so that I could hug my imperfections.

The story of Padma

There was once a woman called Padma, and she lived in a little village in the Dindigul district in the State of Tamil Nadu in India. Each day Padma walked to the watering hole, to collect her water. Across her shoulders she balanced a pole and on either end a terracotta collecting pot was strung. This meant that Padma could carry her water pots safely to the watering hole and return with them full of water. However one of Padma's pots was cracked. She would fill it at the watering hole and then begin her return journey. As Padma walked the water spilled out through the crack and by the time she was home the broken pot was empty while the other was still full. The women in her village laughed at her and ridiculed her for carrying a cracked pot and then filling it with water, day after day.

Padma turned to them and pointed out that beside the path where she walked, there were flowers from wonderful plants and there were insects, butterflies and birds flying around.

Padma went on to say that she continues to take the pot with a crack because even though it has imperfections it is perfect for creating a colourful, fertile piece of ground that the wildlife love. What is imperfect to one person is perfect to another.

Comparison

Comparison is a negative behaviour that reinforces a negative attitude, for example, 'they do this much better than me, and therefore I am not good enough,' which has at its root conformity and competition. As a teacher I was forever comparing myself to younger, more dynamic teachers. As a partner, I was constantly comparing myself to younger women. These comparisons did not support me towards living the best life possible; these comparisons created misery.

I have a strong memory of the experience of comparison from when I was a child. My mum was an amazing knitter. She bought knitting patterns and used them as a basis for her designs. Her jumpers often loosely resembled the picture that was on the front of the pattern, and they often had far more intricate patterns than the one shown. Family, friends, and neighbours all asked my mum to knit them jumpers. She was so quick that she was able to fit their jumpers in around producing a knitted wardrobe for my dad and me. I think my mum invented multi-tasking as she could practically do everything while she was knitting. What I did not discover until much later was that although my mum bought and used knitting patterns, she could not read and write. She hid this fact from most of the world, including me, her only daughter. However, she could design and create the most amazing patterns with a ball of wool and two sticks. I never appreciated my mum's incredible skill.

Growing up I had the most incredible collection of jumpers, gloves, hats, scarves, socks and skirts, all hand knitted. Of course some of these jumpers included jumpers that were a part of my school uniform and needed to be worn to school. My mum would use the fact that I had to wear this jumper to school to showcase her latest design. I would be stood in the middle of a group of my friends' mothers and pulled and poked about as they examined my mum's latest work. As if this was not bad enough, all I ever wanted was a jumper from a store that was plain and knitted on a machine. Then I could be like everyone else. I can remember swapping one of my mother's creations with a girl in my class, just so I could have her 'ordinary' jumper. I was comparing my jumpers with my peers and not liking the answer I came up with. The reason that the answer made me feels unhappy was because I wanted to fit in, and of course in my fancy jumper I stood out. All I wanted to do was hide.

Through the stress of the later years of teaching, my need to compare grew and I think that comparisons stole my happiness. There were times when I went to work and I felt good about my family and myself but in a split second, it would just go. On an either conscious or subconscious level, I began comparing myself with other teachers, and I would find myself falling into the competition and conformity trap, which cultivated my misery.

Blame

During 2008/09/10, I had adopted an attitude to explain that whatever was going on in my life was absolutely nothing to do with me. Something or someone outside of me had caused it. I was not responsible and certainly not to blame. I blamed the government for changing the pension age from 60 to 65; I blamed the weather for making me sit on the sofa and watch TV; I blamed a well-known supermarket for moving onto my doorstep and making me buy wine and chocolate; I blamed everyone in my life for my lethargy. This attitude had serious consequences. If something or somebody, outside of me, was causing all my problems I was therefore powerless and unable to do anything about them. I was a victim and I felt sorry for myself. Blaming others for my situation was perpetuating the trap I was in and led me into an angry downward spiral.

Changing the way I saw things now was top of my list. Blame was not going to change anything. It was going to keep me stuck in the same place. I took a long hard look at my situation and myself and in order to gain some clarity about who I was and where I wanted to go, I decided to use something called the 3Ps and 1W Call to Action. The 3Ps stand for: 1 Problem, 2 Possible causes, 2 Possible solutions. 1W Call to Action means: What's next? My dad discovered the 3P's from reading *How to Win Friends and Influence People* by Dale Carnegie, One of the aims of *How to Win Friends and Influence People* was to get you out of a mental rut, give you new thoughts, new visions, and new ambitions. The 3Ps supports self-exploration of challenges or issues that you may be facing. My dad used the 3Ps often to clarify issues with his brothers and together they added the 1W Call to Action. The 3P's and 1W Call to Action is a strategy I have found that can be used from minor to major issues and challenges whether they are personal or professional. Details of how to carry out 3Ps and 1W are in the Pathway Gems for this chapter.

Challenging my attitude

Writing this book and working with the material and technique of The MACE Pathway, I have had some interesting insights.

My story of my mid-life unravelling is small, insignificant and commonplace. However, our individual stories are about us untangling aspects of our lives and connecting with others. I think our stories shape us, they give us lineage, and a sense of history. Importantly, our stories give us a sense of self. The stories that we have to share about our mid-life are of us being challenged to let go of who we think we are supposed to be and embracing who we are. They are about changing the way we see things. I have shared my story because it is a small story with a big heart and I hope that through my story we have connected. My goal for the future is to inspire and empower children, women and men to change the way they see things now.

I am passionate about *The Time for Freedom* because I hope that it makes a difference. As I sit here and write I am aware that I have not worked in such a focused way for over a year now. I find myself working harder and for longer hours, with more concentrated effort. It is relatively easy because I love creating The Time For Freedom. I have found that if I love what I am doing, work flows. While writing *The Time for Freedom* I have shared my personal story. I have also shared my learning. I really like the fact that some of my story and some of my learning may inspire and empower you to change the way you see things, now. One lesson that has taken me many years to learn is that when I love what I am doing, what I am doing tends to flow out of me easily. It isn't a struggle. On the other hand, when I do not love what I am doing, it seems to exhaust me.

On exploring and examining my life, I discovered that the times when I loved what I did were the happiest times for me. During these times I was focused on what I wanted to create, and loving what I was doing. It was about my attitude of mind. It was the fact that I was living with my Life Purpose in my mind. My Life Purpose is to inspire and empower children, women and men to love trust and believe in themselves so that they change the way they see things now. Writing this book is totally in alignment with my purpose and this makes the work that is generated flow with energy and focus.

Finding self-compassion

We live in an incredibly competitive society. It seems that it is no longer OK to feel good about ourselves, we have to feel outstanding or special or excellent. Anything less seems like failure. I began to accept myself with an open heart and treat myself with the same compassion I would have treated a friend. Actually I would not have treated a stranger the way I had been treating myself. I think it is important that we accept ourselves totally. There is only one antidote to this problem and this simply is self-acceptance. This is a major step towards peace of mind, accepting yourself as you are now, unconditionally. Self-compassion is defined in one dictionary as 'being open to, and moved by one's own suffering, experiencing feeling of caring and kindness towards oneself, taking an understanding, non-judgemental attitude toward one's inadequacies and failures, and recognising that one's experiences are part of the common human experience'. Sometimes we are our own worst enemies!

I have shared self-compassion at my workshops and with friends and colleagues. Some participants, friends and colleagues thought that self-compassion was a form of self-pity, and others thought it was a dressed up word for self-indulgence. I wanted to dispel the notion that a focus on self-compassion did not mean that my problems are more important than yours; it just means that I think that my problems are also important and worthy of being attended to. I wanted them to see that self-compassion involves wanting health and wellbeing for oneself and leads to proactive behaviour to betters one's situation, rather than passivity. I learnt through reading and talking to people that rather than condemning myself for my mistakes and failures, I could use the experience to soften my heart and let go of those harsh unrealistic expectations of perfection that had made me so dissatisfied. The door blew open to real and lasting satisfaction just by giving myself the compassion I needed in the moment. Self-compassion is very important, not only because it encourages us to be kinder to ourselves, but also some of us are harsh on ourselves because we believe that if we celebrate ourselves or if we are kind to ourselves it is a form of narcissism.

Self-compassion is especially important when we 'fail' at things in life, which is inevitable. It is a part of normal human experience. If we are self-compassionate and apply strategies for being compassionate to ourselves, it is possible to recover from disappointment and to find positive ways of interpreting difficult experiences and seeing something of value in them. Kindness towards ourselves is very important, and is caring for our own needs. When we take care of ourselves, we begin to expand. We have more energy, confidence, wisdom and clarity. Be kind to yourself.

From: Do Be Have to Be Do Have

For most of my life the attitude that I had adopted which had motivated me and had underpinned my life was:

DO   – I am going to do something to make some money.

BE   – I will be able to do what I want to do.

HAVE – I will have happiness and success.

My life had embraced the above. In today's society, it is the conventional model of how to live life. It is replicated in films, on TV, in stories and magazines. If we are to be happy and successful we go to work to earn money to buy things or do things that make us happy. This is exactly what I was doing. I was climbing the career ladder of teaching, no matter how many hours of work it generated or the level of stress it created in me just so that I would earn more money to eventually make me happy.

I wondered about our search for happiness and success. Have you ever asked yourself why you are doing what you are doing? Why you are in your job? Why you want to make money? While writing this book I spoke to many people about these questions. It seems the overriding reason we go to work is provide us with money and things to make us happy. In fact life has become one big never-ending pursuit of contented feelings that can only be satisfied through external stimulus. It is interesting but this search for inner contentment and happiness seems to be universal. Although we pursue happiness, we are not happy!

A Story: The Musk Deer

There is a species of deer that produces musk in its own body. When it begins to smell the musk, the deer yearns for the musk and so begins searching endlessly for the source of this aroma. The musk smell mesmerises the deer. It searches and forages for the smell but cannot find it. What the deer of course does not realise is that it is the source of the very thing that it is searching for. It is lying within itself.

I felt a lot like the deer in the story and it resonated with me deeply. The deer had everything that it needed and yet it was in search of something outside of itself to make it feel okay. The deer in the story is living a life of Do Be Have. A life of looking outside of themselves.

I wanted to change the way I saw things and begin to live it as Be-Do-Have.

- Be: who you need to be.
- Do: in order to do what you need to do.
- Have: to have what you want to achieve.

Our human dilemma is just like that, we seek the answers outside of ourselves, without realising that what we seek, happiness, love and wisdom, already lies within us. When we are children, we learn to stop looking to ourselves to know what is right for us. Instead of trusting our intuitive knowledge, we turn to others. First we look to our parents and then to our teachers, friends, partner and children. We assume that the love, the acceptance, and the approval are out there and that we must earn it in some way. The answers are within us.

Conclusion

Believing in ourselves is at the heart of The MACE Pathway: ATTITUDE. This is not always easy to carry out when for much of our lives we have been taught that there is something wrong with us or that we are imperfect. When we allow negative thoughts and feelings to flood our hearts and minds on a constant basis they betray our inner majesty. This is an illusion and we are all perfect and I began to change the way I saw things. We have all been given the power of choice to choose in each moment how we want to 'Be'; whether to be happy or sad, clear or confused, full of inspiration or depressed. We always have the choice either to despise and wound others or to be kind and respectful to them.

We have the ability to believe in hope and faith as opposed to hopelessness and doubt. Hope is a way of thinking. Emotions have a role to play with hope, however hope is a cognitive process that happens when:

- I know where I want to go.
- I know how to get there and I will persist and tolerate disappointment.
- I know that I can do this.

We are all loveable, capable and significant.

Pathway Gems

Captured Thoughts:

'Nobody sees a flower – really – it is so small,
it takes time – we haven't time – and to see takes time,
like to have a friend takes time.'

Georgia O'Keeffe

'If you think adventure is dangerous, try routine, it is lethal.'

Paul Coelho, author

Movement, Action, Creativity and Enjoyment

Movement – Mirror Twist

- Lower your arms in front to shoulder height, palms facing away, fingers pointing upwards and elbows slightly bent. Keep your knees soft.

- Turn your right palm so that it is facing towards you. Keeping your left hand where it is, move your right arm around to the right as you twist your spine.

- Focus on the palm of your right hand as if looking in a mirror and say out loud 'Hello Gorgeous!' And acknowledge yourself.

- Pause.

- Slowly reverse the movement and come to face the front again.

- Reverse the position of your palms and repeat on the left side.

- Relax your arms down.
- Once you have practised these movements incorporate the breath as follows:
    - Breathe out as you twist.
    - Hold as you pause in the extended position.
    - Breathe in as you return to the front.

Action – The 3Ps and 1W

1. Identify and write down one Problem or challenge.
2. Write down Possible causes of the problem or challenge.
3. Write down Possible solutions to the problem or challenge.
4. Ask yourself What's next?

Record your experience, insights and outcomes, drawing or writing, using any colour pen or pencil, in your journal.

Action – Gratitude

If you find yourself glued to negative emotions and don't know how to get yourself out then STOP thinking about how much you are stuck in the emotion – you are simply entrenching that habit more and more deeply. The key here is to start with gratitude.

- Sit comfortably in a quiet space. If you want you can light a candle, whatever you can do to take you into your own space – ideally shut the door and turn off the phone.
- Think of someone you deeply love – this can be yourself, a partner, a child, a friend or a member of your family. For these exercises choose someone you have a personal relationship with.
- Really start to feel your love of that person in your heart. Feel it growing and becoming stronger – almost as if you are turning up the volume.

- Allow that feeling of love to change subtly so that you start to appreciate everything about the person: their physical appearance, their personality, and the joy you feel in their presence. Allow appreciation to become a deeper feeling still as it turns into gratitude that the person is a part of your life. Again really feel the quality of gratitude as you focus on that person.

- Start to turn that feeling of gratitude inwards now, towards who YOU really are. Start to appreciate and love things about yourself, just as you do about the other person. Hold a sense of gratitude that you are here on this earth, that you are living a wonderful life, that you have a fantastic body that carries you everywhere. Recognise that, in reality, you have everything that you need. Right here and now.

- When you are ready, slowly bring yourself back into the present moment, but if you can, hold on to that feeling of deep peace and appreciation.

I hope that this short concentration technique will help you to become more focused on the amazing being that you are so that you step out with confidence and bring strength into your life. Know that you are fantastic just as you are. Once you have that under your belt then we can start with directing those emotions to bring even greater joy and success to your life.

Action – An Exploration of Self-Compassion

One day I wrote down all the things I did not like about myself. All the things that cause me shame or make me feel insecure; that I'm not good enough. I focused on how I looked physically, my appearance, my behaviour at work, at home, socially, my relationship, any issues that I thought I had.

When I had all the above on paper, I began to write down how all this made me feel. Words like 'scared, depressed, angry, bored, insecure, miserable,' flew onto the page.

I put the piece of paper to one side.

I then called to mind an imaginary friend who unconditionally loves me, who is accepting, kind and compassionate. I imagined that this friend could see all my strengths and all my weaknesses, including all that I had written down. I thought about how this friend might feel towards me. How this friend loved me just the way I was with all my human imperfections. My imaginary friend was kind and forgiving and recognised the limitations of human nature. She also had great wisdom and understood my life history.

I gave this imaginary friend a name. I called her Sylvia.

I then wrote a letter to myself from Sylvia. I focused on what Sylvia would say to me about all my self-conceived flaws. I wrote compassionately and reminded myself about being only human and that we all have strengths and weaknesses. In the letter Sylvia also told me about unconditional understanding and compassion.

As I wrote I infused the letter with a strong sense of personal acceptance, kindness, caring and desire for my health and happiness.

I put the letter down and went for a short walk. When I returned I re-read the letter, letting the words sink deep inside me. I could feel the compassion pour into me, soothing and comforting me. In that instant I learnt that love, connection and acceptance are my birth right, and to claim them I only need to look inside myself.

I invite you to write a self-compassion letter to yourself.

Creativity – capturing your whispers

I invite you to use all or some of these prompts and record your responses in whatever creative way you choose.

- What can you learn from stories?
- What is your story?
- Creative expression is contagious and loves company.
- Stories keep the delicious details alive and flavour the facts.
- Let your stories tumble out.

Enjoyment is about having fun along the way. Not worrying about what others may think, feel, say or do. It is about your nourishment. Do what you need to do today to bring Enjoyment into your life.

Chapter 3
THE MACE PATHWAY: COMMITMENT

Remember, The MACE Pathway is a spiral pathway, upwards to the top of the most majestic, powerful and ancient mountain. Your mountain. While walking on the earth pathway, The MACE Pathway takes you around so you can view with a critical eye all of your thoughts, beliefs, attitudes, habits, life's experiences and views. Walking the steady trail and reaching the top is about reaching your dream. Sometimes we dream and then we have to dare ourselves to do. COMMITMENT – A Call To Action is reminding ourselves that we have the choice to dream and it is our action that creates our futures.

Applying The MACE Pathway to my life and reaching the top of my mountain was about me successfully realising my dream. My dream was to write a book that would inspire and empower its readers to change the way they saw things.

Dream Dare Do!

For many years of my life I went from day to day completing routines at work and at home. My life was dull. In 2010 I got my wakeup call and I heard it, loud and clear. I decided that it was time that I committed to my dream. My dream was to publish a book that would make a difference and *The Time for Freedom* is that book. I dared to do the things that I felt were missing in my life. In 2010 the main reason that kept me stuck and unable to move was my belief that that my life had passed me by. I had given up on myself and felt that I was too old to have dreams and to action them. Oh my goodness, I am so very grateful to John and his question and the thump it gave me.

In 1994 I had a dream and a dream is just a goal without a deadline. I had this dream that I was so passionate about that I shared it, I talked about it, I nurtured it, I loved it and I gave it heaps of attention and resources over the years. I wanted to write a book that would inspire and empower its readers to love, trust and believe in themselves and change the way they saw things so that they could live a great life. It has taken me a good few years to write. But I write today, from love and wisdom and *The Time for Freedom* is my dream come true. It may have been a long gap between 1994 and 2012, however this time it is perfect! My journey, learning and action to manifesting *The Time for Freedom* has been one of incredible insight.

Although I had a dream to write a book, I had a strong belief that I was not a good enough writer to carry out the task. I have learnt through experience that we <u>learn the most about ourselves when we do the thing we never thought we could do</u>. This is a very important sentence. Please read the underlined section again. It is when we do what we think we cannot do, that we unearth our potential and extend our limits. Our inner whispers get nurtured and our spirits soar. I did not believe that I could leave teaching and become a published author. I thought my life would fall apart.

When we do the things we didn't think we could do, something shifts inside us. We push our boundaries. We find strength in ourselves that we didn't know was there. When we push our boundaries without intending to do so we shed layers of perfectionism, worry, fear and self-doubt. Underneath all these layers I discovered, exists our creativity.

My journey in writing *The Time for Freedom* taught me the invaluable life-changing lesson that anything is possible in our lives when we change the way we see things.

Listen to your whispers

Paying attention to our inner whispers is one of the most exciting and loving things that we can do for ourselves. Sometimes we cover our whispers so that we cannot hear or see them because we are feeling limited by decisions we've already made in our lives. We fear change and so do not give ourselves permission to change, to evolve. Commit to listening to your inner whispers.

These whispers are the seeds of your dream. Follow them to their truth. This may mean that you do the thing that scares you the most, discovering your buried dreams. Commit to dreaming, daring and doing. It is about you rediscovering your worth and your potential and inspiring and empowering you to fly on their wings.

Do you have a voice inside, a gentle whisper quietly nudging you to listen? What does it say? Those internal whispers tug at us and want our attention. The whispers are the seeds of our dreams. Our whispers tend to reveal themselves someplace where they know they are safe. Your journal is such a good place to capture and find them. Sometimes our whispers pop up within an inner dialogue during quiet moments. Sometimes when I am on a bus or waiting for a train, or soaking in the bath, my mind begins to dream. Some call this daydreaming. I believe the daydreams are whispers, disguised because they tend to give me new ideas, plans and dreams. There are times when our inner whispers become visible or audible as they thread across emails, texts, telephone conversations or letters to friends, loved ones and family. Amongst the words sometimes there is a clue, 'if I had more time I would… one day maybe I can…' Take time to notice your whispers.

From time to time the constraints and pressures of our everyday lives suffocate our dream whispers. That is exactly what happened to me until 2010. I had no idea what my dreams were, and because I was not conscientious about the presence of my dreams in my life, then they were buried underneath the layers of everyday detail: teaching, cleaning the house, shopping, planning holidays. Each day came and went, and there I was fifty-eight years old, with the possibility of only 17 years left and a pocket full of dreams that had been neglected and were covered over with layers of life. I became aware that my inner yearnings were my living dreams. I also realised that my dreams were my life's possibility for today. I had woken up and I wondered who I was, what were my passions, what were my dreams for my life and where did they all go?

What is commitment?

If you should be wondering what is commitment, a good way to find out would be to put your head underwater and keep it there for a while. You'll soon realise that you're 100 per cent committed to breathing and get your head out of the water! Do notice though:

- You didn't make excuses not to breathe.
- You didn't worry about motivating yourself to breathe.
- You didn't need to justify your desire to breathe.
- A clear intention began to form within a matter of seconds.
- You were soon breathing.

A commitment to 'breathe' happened in a heartbeat! The urgency I felt from John's question, when I saw 17 years flashing in front of me, was a loud and resounding Call to Action. I told myself I did not have time for:

- Excuses.
- Debate.
- Lengthy analysis.
- Moaning about how hard it is.
- Worrying about what others might think.
- Delays.
- Worrying about scarce resources.

Turning a dream into a goal is a powerful process for committing to your future. A commitment to create your best life. It is about listening to your whispers, reading your captured whispers and turning your vision of your future into reality, all within a frame of time. The process of setting goals helps you choose and commit to where you want to go in life. By knowing your dreams, daring to concentrate your efforts and doing all you can to spot the distractions that can so easily lead you off course.

Not having a goal is like attempting to sail a boat without a rudder. It is essential for direction. If you are sailing a boat and you do not have a rudder you are likely to be blown around by the wind and waves.

If we do not unearth our goals and commit to them, we could be on our deathbeds and not have dreamed, dared or done! Our lives are important. Listen and capture your whispers so that you have a long-term vision and are motivated. Having a goal also supports you in organising your time, gathering resources and being clear about your acquisition of knowledge. This all helps you make the most of your life.

Setting sharp, clearly defined goals and moving towards them using baby steps will raise your self-confidence as you recognise your own ability and competence. I have set goals for myself, empowered others to set goals and talked widely about the importance of goal setting and goal getting. I believe that when we set ourselves a goal and put our dream out in the world, we line ourselves, our resources and our focus up behind it. As we move towards our goal one step at a time, our confidence and self-esteem grows. With success comes self-belief. This whole process is developmentally good for us.

Why set goals?

- Goals can focus you to work towards something.

- Each day we set goals. We get out of bed and we begin our day. That is in itself is a goal. We may have a To Do list and this is a list of goals. If you were to plan a holiday that would be a goal. Our subconscious mind helps us seek our goals. We need to make sure that we give

81

our subconscious our goals, otherwise it will pursue targets that we may not necessarily have chosen. For example, worrying about something sends a negative message or negative goal to our subconscious. Clear goals about what is most important, supports, and gives a strong message to our subconscious about how to move forward.

- Goals can help you concentrate your time and effort.

- One reason why people who set goals have success in their lives is because they have learned how to focus and concentrate their time, energy and resources on a single objective, even if it is just for a few hours at a time. Their powers of concentration can produce results that are much greater than those achievable through the diffused and unfocused energy many people use to get through their days. One major issue for many of us today, tends to be time management and it is very easy to diffuse our time and energy with many different pursuits, aimless distractions and general busyness. Goals provide a way to focus and concentrate your time and energy into carefully chosen targets. Goals are designed to make significant positive impacts in your life.

- Goals can provide motivation, persistence, and desire.

- Our most significant accomplishments are riddled with obstacles, struggles, and failures. It is estimated that Thomas Edison failed over one thousand times before he finally discovered a way to make the light bulb work. It is very rare for something important to be accomplished successfully on the very first try.

- If you want to achieve anything, it is likely that you will struggle and fail many times before you finally reach your goal. Goal setters pick themselves up after each fall and continue working steadily towards their targets until they finally reach their goal. Struggle and failure are often part of the price that we have to pay for our achievements.

- Goals can help you establish priorities.

- There will be many forks in the road between where you are now and where you want to be. Instead of just letting the 'current' or other people's interests determine where you end up, you have to consciously decide which way to go. Goals and the dreams that inspired them provide a natural framework to help you identify and establish your priorities and make the 'right' choices.

- Goals can provide a map to take you from where you are to where you want to be.

- Setting a clear and well-intentioned goal is good to get you on your way. However it helps to have sub-goals that help you with stepping-stones towards your main goal. Sub-goals give you valuable feedback, they tell you whether you are making progress or not and can warn you if you are getting off course.

Stop. Look. Take action!

In almost any goal or project you will need to make adjustments to your goals and plans. You will need to take risks, make mistakes and learn from them.

A question of time

The timing issue is the one that trips us up and prevents us from enjoying and achieving our goals. Sometimes when we consider a particular goal we worry about a time commitment and put a time challenge in the way, such as:

- I'm so overweight it could take years to get into shape.

- If I break off this unfulfilling relationship, it could take years to get back on my feet again.

- If I start my own business now it could take years to make a profit.

- Even if start writing now, I will never finish my book.

- I am so unhealthy it will take me months to get back to being healthy.

- It took 20 years to make me this ill, it will take me another 20 to get well.

This self-talk reveals a misunderstanding of time. There is an understanding that time is a resource that we spend in the same way that we spend money. For example, to complete a one-hour task is to spend an hour on it. How are you 'spending' your day? Where do you want to 'spend' the weekend? How will you 'spend' your retirement? Time seems to be a disposable resource – after all time is money, isn't it? I think time is not a resource. I do not believe that you can spend time. Time will spend itself. We have no choice in the matter. No matter what I do in the next 10 minutes, time will move on. It doesn't matter if I do nothing or something for the next five years. Those five years will pass whatever I do.

In reality, we are never in our past or in our future. We only exist in the present moment. Even when you or I remember our past, or envisage our future, we are still thinking those thoughts from our present moment. All we have is right now, and that is all we will ever have. We cannot control time. We can control how we are being in our present moment. That's all. Just right now.

Setting a goal is not about the future: it brings clarity here and now.

If we accept that we can only achieve anything in the present moment, and that you can only enjoy those achievements in the present moment, it is not possible to enjoy anything in the past or future because we are not there.

The important point to remember about setting goals is that it improves the quality of our present moment reality. Setting a goal can give us greater clarity and focus right now. Whenever we set a goal it is important to check in with ourselves and ask the question, how does setting this goal improve my present reality? If a goal does not improve your present reality, then the goal is pointless and you may as well put it in the bin. But if your goal brings greater clarity, focus and motivation to your life whenever you think about it, then it is something to keep to.

Some of us set goals and then assume the path to reach them will be arduous and strenuous and will involve suffering and sacrifice. That is a clear recipe for failure. Another approach would be to set a goal and consider how it is affecting your present moments. The important point is to set goals that have a positive effect on your life whenever you think about them. This is important long before the final outcome is arrived at. I think that goal setting is a way to boost each day and add to present reality, rather than a way to control the future.

Here is an example:

- You would like to start your own business, so you set your goal to start your own business.
- You can see yourself at some time in the future, doing what you love and making a great income.

Nothing wrong with that. What drifts into your mind though is how much work it will take, the risks you will face and many other demotivating and discouraging thoughts. You are no longer in the present. You have moved to the future, which is not happening. You are just making it up, a story in fact. Why do we make things up, that we do not want?

Looking at this differently?

- You would like to start your own business, so you set your goal to start your own business.

- You imagine how great it is, everything is running smoothly.

Staying present in the present moment. Consider how this goal could improve the quality of your life right now. Not in the future, not tomorrow, next week, next month, next year. How could this business improve your life right now? What does this goal of your own business do for you here and now? What does it give you? Hope? Does it inspire you? Does it come with any promises? Let those thoughts move through you. Consider how the goal of starting your own business improves your life right now. If you set yourself a goal and you cannot see it improving your life here and now, then it is time to consider another goal.

If I had not brought imaginary obstacles into my path I might have set goals earlier around leaving my teaching post and enjoying a more fulfilling career. What stopped me setting those goals towards leaving my teaching post was the fact that all I saw was doom, gloom, insecurity and scarcity of resources. When I stopped thinking about my goal being in the future and I brought it into my present I immediately became motivated to take action. And coincidentally I began attracting resources into my life that supported me towards achieving my goal. I did not have to force myself, I found myself naturally drawn to take action as I kept bringing my focus back to my present. When I thought about my goal in this way, I was motivated to take action in alignment with that goal. From this perspective if you set goals to increase the quality of your present reality, time is no longer the major factor – having fun and feeling fulfilled takes precedence along the way. Also when you focus on each day as taking you towards your goal, you begin to feel happy and fulfilled. And this drives you to take enjoyable action and boosts your productivity.

Whatever goal you set for yourself, you have the choice of looking towards your future and deciding which approach towards your goal that you will take: one approach which will create sacrifice and suffering or, another which focuses on today and the present reality with new hope, enthusiasm and motivation. Even though the goals are set for the future they are also set for today. This is such an important point for being able to attain successful goals. Make sure that the goal you are working for is something that you really want, not just something that sounds good or that someone else has thought up as a good idea. Successful goal setting and getting operates with the fundamental principle of owning your own goal. With that ownership comes the enjoyment of the journey of and towards your goal.

How does positive thinking affect our goal getting?

We have 12,000 to 50,000 thoughts a day. Most of them are repetitive and are about routine tasks that we carry out every day but there are plenty of others that come from our internal self-talk. Do you know what are you telling yourself day after day? Do you have positive thoughts and use encouraging words that are helping you towards your dreams and goals, or negative, unhelpful thoughts?

I'm sure you have heard many times already that we should think positively. And you may think that sometimes it is just ridiculous, how can you be positive when you are unhappy with your life, living in poverty, working in a dead end job and a living a stressful life. It is worth taking a moment to consider the message that you are sending repeatedly to your subconscious mind. The more you think negatively about your life, work, family etc., the stronger and clearer the message.

Your conscious mind is responsible for judgement, strategy, and making decisions in your life. Our subconscious mind does what it is told to do by our conscious mind. Our subconscious is not judging what is good or bad, it assumes you know best. Your subconscious is your 'genie' and will bring to you what you ask it for. It works twenty-four hours a day, and oversees your body's systems, habits, any learnt skills and your behaviour. Science continues to be mystified by the power of the human subconscious.

Conscious and sub-conscious mind

Knowing about the role of our conscious and subconscious mind is important for us when it comes to us wanting to successfully achieve our goals.

A story: The Peacock and the Elephant

In ancient times the conscious mind was likened to a peacock because of its tendency to display itself and make a loud and raucous noise. The subconscious mind was likened to an elephant because it is quiet, huge, remembers everything, and is difficult to get to move unless you have its trust and it actually wants to move. When it does move though, it is unstoppable, and if it becomes enraged, then everyone gets out of its way.

Our subconscious mind acts on the information that the conscious mind gives it. We know that there is a subconscious mind because of the effects that it has on the conscious mind. All of us know that there is more than the conscious mind, and that the subconscious mind can be our greatest ally or worst enemy. If we do not set a goal, then our subconscious seeks our dominant thoughts and uses them as commands. Therefore, whatever you think about, good, bad or indifferent becomes a goal command for your subconscious to manifest. Therefore, when we worry we set a negative goal. Worrying about what we don't want, or fear, is like setting a negative goal. That is the up and down side to the subconscious. Sometimes we think we are asking for one thing, and we get another. Your subconscious mind filters out anything that is irrelevant to what you asked it to provide.

Good examples of our subconscious in action is when we walk to the shops, take the school run or drive to a familiar destination. Sometimes we can arrive and we hardly remember walking or driving there. This is because your subconscious was walking or driving for you. Whatever you bring into your focus and work towards becomes a goal for your subconscious to pursue. Keeping our subconscious focused on what we want to create in our lives is important for our success. Giving our subconscious commands that we want it to work on supports us in maximising our potential.

Positive thoughts can affect our self-belief. I have a friend called Dorothy who has a serious illness that affects her spine. According to medical practitioners, Dorothy should be in a wheelchair. However Dorothy regularly walks, she has a daily yoga session and hardly ever uses the lift in a building or takes the bus into town. According to specialists at the local hospital, she is a miracle. I spoke with Dorothy and asked about her situation.

Dorothy talked about her days of living each day in a wheelchair and her commitment to herself to begin her journey to start walking again. Dorothy believed that she could walk and she talked to herself positively each day. Although she was unable to walk, she visualised herself practising yoga and walking each day.

The belief that Dorothy held about herself was powerful, and had a huge effect on her mentally, emotionally and physically. Her beliefs sent a strong, clear and focused command to her subconscious about what was important to her, and what she wanted. Each day Dorothy held her belief and it got stronger and stronger. Each day her self-belief became deeper and deeper, positively affecting her habits and patterns. Repeated thoughts accepted as true become beliefs, feelings become attitudes actions become habits.

We can see from Dorothy's story that self-belief can be incredibly powerful, especially when we set a goal that we believe in.

Our thoughts affect our thinking

Scientists in the past used to believe that we responded to information flowing into the brain. However today, more and more evidence is being collected that is telling us that we respond to what the brain expects to happen next on the basis of previous experience. There was a study in the USA involving arthroscopic knee surgery. A group of patients with sore, worn-out knees were assigned to one of three surgical procedures: scraping out the knee joint, washing out the knee joint or doing nothing. During the 'pretend' operation, doctors anaesthetised the patients, made three incisions in the knee as if to insert their surgical instruments, and pretended to operate. Two years after surgery patients who completed the 'pretend' surgery, reported the same amount of relief from pain and swelling as those who had received the actual treatments. The brain expected the 'surgery' to improve the knee, and it did.

Through a lifetime of events and experiences, our brain actually learns what to expect next, whether it eventually happens that way or not. This is the most important point, and because our brain expects something will happen a certain way, we often achieve exactly what we anticipate. This is why it is very important to hold positive expectations in our minds. Believing that what you want is possible gives your brain the signal and it takes over the job of accomplishing that possibility.

When I look back and see myself as I was in 2010, I see a woman who did not believe in herself. My wake up call, gave me the kick I needed. I was able to see that I was capable of changing the way I saw things and making my dreams happen. I was able to believe in myself. It really doesn't matter what title we use, self-assurance, self-confidence, or self-esteem. The result is a deep-seated belief that I have what it takes, the abilities, the inner resources, talents and skills to create my desired results. I learnt that believing in myself is a choice. Over time I learnt that taking responsibility for my attitude develops over time. It is important to remember that when we act as if it is possible then it becomes possible. If you believe that something is impossible then it will be impossible and you will not produce the results that you want. It is a self-fulfilling prophecy. What I wanted to do with my life began with me. I did not ask another's permission. I decided that having others believing in me and my dream was not a requirement for my success. If I was going to have to wait for others to believe in me before I left my work, I would not have accomplished anything. I based my decisions about what I wanted to do on my goals and my desires. Not the goals, desires, opinions, and judgments of my employer, colleagues, family or friends. I stopped worrying what other people thought of me and I followed my heart.

Making that commitment to your goal

Having unearthed your dreams and become clear about your true needs and desires the next steps are for you to sort them and convert them into goals that you are able to act upon with certainty, knowing that you will commit to achieve them. Goal setting is like a muscle and like any muscle the more that it is used the stronger it gets. However, this development has to be paced and gradual. Below are some important points to remember when committing to your goals; they have not been listed in any particular order of importance:

- Act As If. One of the best strategies for bringing your goal to action is to act as if you are already where you want to be. This means thinking like, talking like, dressing like, acting like and feeling like the person who has already achieved their goal. Acting as if sends a powerful command to your subconscious mind to find creative strategies to achieve the goal you are aiming at. It programmes your nervous system in your brain to start noticing anything that will help you succeed and it sends strong messages to your world that this is something that you want.

- Be. Do. Have. It is possible to Act As If, right now. Acting as if you have already achieved any of your goals means being it, doing it and having it. Acting as if as an outer experience will create the inner experience. Acting as if will take you to the actual manifestation of that experience. Deciding as if you already are being, doing, or having your goal.

- Start now. How would you like to think, talk, act, carry yourself, dress, treat other people, handle money, eat, live, travel etc., When you have a clear picture, start being it – now! Start now and be who you want to be, then do the actions that go along with being that person, and soon you will find that you have reached your goal.

- Send a confident message to your subconscious: by believing in your goal and believing in yourself. The more you believe in yourself and your goal the stronger the message to your subconscious.

- Personal Goals. It is important that your goals are about your life and you. You are the only person who can set goals for you. It is not possible to set goals for anyone else and no one else can set goals for you.

- How Much By When. To involve my subconscious my goal need to be stated in such a way that it could be measured and have an end date. The more detail that can be included in your goals always give your subconscious more information to work with. Without the detail, criteria or measurement your goal is not a goal. It is a wish. A wish does not engage your subconscious. And, your subconscious is your friend and more – it is your genie. We have this amazing resource to support us in making our dreams come true and yet we tend not to use it to its maximum potential.

- Write out your goal in detail. I use Brian Mayne's *Goal Mapping The Practical Workbook* for setting my Goals. However, before I put anything on a Goal Map I write out my goal in absolute detail. Writing my goal out in detail gives me clarity. I think of it as a request to myself. If I do not include all the details then how do I know what I want? When you write down all the details your subconscious mind knows what to work on. It will know which opportunities to focus on to help get you closer to your goal.

- Write down your goal using present tense. Your subconscious operates in the present moment and needs goal commands that are set in the present tense.

- Think about goals that stretch you a little. I set goals about my home, planning holidays etc., I also like to write down a goal or two that are Big Hairy Audacious goals that I know will stretch me and maybe make me feel uncomfortable. I know that through these goals, I will develop personally, because the real end result of Goal Setting is not just the goal. It is more than that. When the goal is complete you will have become a leader of your own life. Along this path you will need to learn new skills, be open to possibilities, build new relationships and learn to overcome your fears.

Some reasons that can stop us from successful goal getting

As I talked to people about their lives and their commitments, I also asked them if they didn't set goals, what prevented them and what were their reasons. Here are some of them:

- Some people said that they do not have a good reason to set goals. During our conversation, I pointed out that goals can help you get what you want, but they won't help you figure out what that is! It is important to be clear about what you really want before you set a goal for yourself.

- Some people talked about not knowing about the power of goal setting. Their only knowledge was about theirs and others failed New Year Resolutions. These people did not realise that there was power and value in goal setting and that it could be used as a tool for success. I strongly believe that goal setting should be a part of the school curriculum as it is an amazing self-empowerment tool.

- Others were unsure as to how to use the power of their goals. The common misunderstanding here was that some of these people thought goals were wishes and thought that a goal was something wide and unattainable. In fact something to make fun of.

- Some people were afraid. Fear is a powerful emotion that can be helpful but can also be destructive and paralysing. Goal setting often requires us to overcome several deep-rooted fears: fear of failure, fear of rejection, and fear of the unknown.

- One other reason that people have shared with me as to why they do not set goals is that they are too busy to even consider a new challenge. I have heard many times 'I'll set a goal someday when things settle down a bit and I get a bit more time.' I certainly know what it is like to feel far too stressed and overwhelmed to cope with day-to-day demands.

Goal Mapping

Throughout my life I have set goals. But in 2010, I decided that I wanted a new and fresh approach and I began reading and applying the work of Brian Mayne of LIFT International. Brian and his wife

94

Sangeeta work to help people of all ages evolve and improve their lives. Their organisation LIFT International was founded on the following statement: 'We are a community of *LIFT leaders*. LIFT is *Life Information For Transcendence*. We share Life Information For Transcendence in order to serve the evolution of humanity.' Brian's approach, I felt was in alignment with who I am. *Brian Mayne's Goal Mapping* is a unique whole-brain system designed to connect your consciously chosen goals to your subconscious mind so that your subconscious begins to automatically move you and your goal towards each other.

Goal Mapping uses both sides of our brain to support us in attaining our goals. We all have two sides to our brains, which operate somewhat independently of one another, which means we all do not think the same way. Some of us have a preference for verbal thinking, step by step reasoning, taking a logical, mathematical approach which is associated with the left side of the brain, and others think non-verbally, creatively, musically, mystically using the right side of their brain. We live in a left brain dominant world and many of us operate more from the rational left brain, which tends to override the creativity and originality of the right brain. No one is totally left brained or totally right brained. Just as you have a dominant hand, dominant eye and even a dominant foot, you probably also have a dominant side of your brain. An understanding of our preferred way of thinking and learning can help us to maintain successful relationships and balanced lifestyles. Knowing how we think is useful, because when we want to plan, organise or set goals we learn to stimulate our left brain patterns and if we want to relax, be more intuitive and creative or have more peaceful thoughts, we need to operate our right brain.

Brian Mayne's Goal Mapping system uses both left and right brain. His Goal Map template helped me organise, plan and write my goals, which stimulated my left-brain patterns. With my Goal Map I also used the right side of my brain, which is more intuitive and creative, by using pictures and diagrams and symbols. Please see my own Goal Map on the following pages.

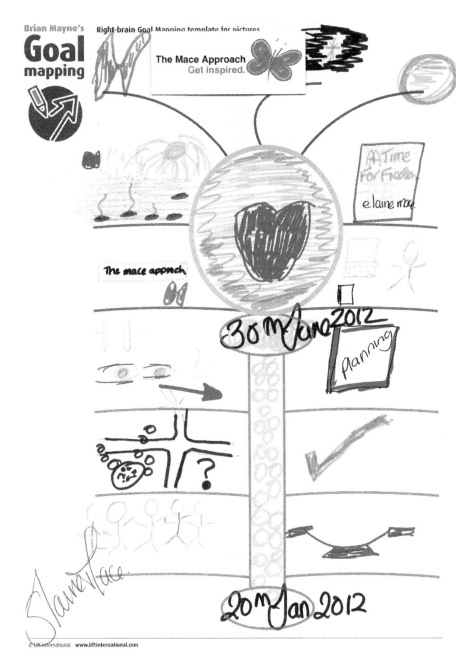

These pages show my personal Goal Maps, covering the period from January to June 2012.

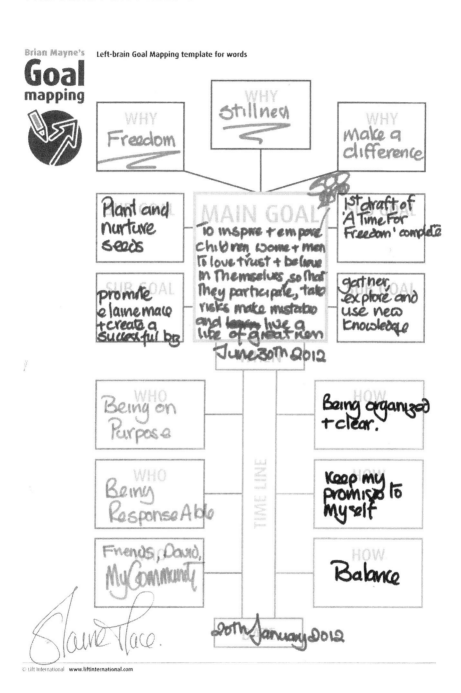

Since attending a LIFT International Goal Mapping Workshop I have qualified as a Goal Mapping Practitioner and I run inspirational and empowering Success Workshops for adults, young people and children. You can find out more information about my work from my website elainemace.com. To find out more about Brian Mayne's work and LIFT International visit liftinternational.com.

Bringing my goals alive!

I have my Goal Map on my wall in front of where I work each day. Before I begin work in the morning, I spend some time absorbing my goal map. Reflecting on what it means to me, by carrying out the following practice:

1. By looking at my Map, I reinforce the commands to my subconscious. This helps me control any sneaky bits of self-doubt that may have crept into my mind. In addition, visualising my Goal Map activates the right side of my brain and supports me with vision.

2. After looking at my Goal Map, I read it out loud. This activates the left side of my brain and supports me in planning and prioritising.

3. I take a few more minutes to commit to at least five things that I will carry out during that day that will be taking me closer to my goal. These are my baby steps.

This practice supports me in connecting with my Goal Map. It reminds me what is important in my life. It also gives me vital information about what I need to do today to take me closer to manifesting my dream.

Conclusion

The MACE Pathway: COMMITMENT is most definitely a Call To Action. A time to take some time to unearth your dreams, acknowledge them and to commit to them becoming a part of your life. You can make this happen in a heartbeat.

Pathway Gems

Captured Thoughts:

'Do one thing every day that scares you.'

> Eleanor Roosevelt, First Lady of the United States from 1933 to 1945

'If you want it go for it, take a risk don't always play it safe or you'll die wondering.'

> Exceptional Living (facebook.com/MyExceptionalLiving)

'I want to be thoroughly used up when I die, for the harder I work the more I live. I rejoice in life for its own sake. Life is no "brief candle" for me. It is a sort of splendid torch which I have got hold of for the moment, and I want to make it burn as brightly as possible before handing it on to future generations.'

> George Bernard Shaw, Playwright

Movement, Action, Creativity and Enjoyment

Movement – Dru Yoga – The Archer

The Archer is a great posture to support you as you work towards your goal or dream.

- Adjust your feet to two shoulder-widths apart.
- Turn your right foot out 90 degrees to the right and push your left heel back slightly so that your right heel is in line with the instep of your left foot. Imagine that you are an archer ready to draw your bow as follows:

- Stretch your right hand out to the right with your palm pushing away and fingers pointing up.

- Bring your left hand in front of your chest, with your thumb up and your forefinger and middle fingers extended and the ring and little fingers tucked into the palm of your hand.

- Stand with your weight balanced equally on both feet and your hips facing forwards.

- Breathe in and draw your left hand across your chest towards your left shoulder, keeping your arm at shoulder height.

- Feel the stretch between your arms as you create the necessary tension to release your arrow.

- As you draw the bowstring towards your ear, transfer your weight onto your left foot beginning at the knee.

- Pause for a moment and visualise your goal.

- Breathe out and release the arrow letting it fly towards your goal.

- As it does so transfer your weight from the left leg onto the right leg, bending your right knee and turning your body to face right.

- Gently sweep your arms in front of your body, pivot your feet to face the opposite direction and repeat on the other side.

Action – Are you Right- or Left-Brained?

Answer yes or no to the following questions:

1. Are you a list maker?

2. Do you enjoy making schedules and daily planning?

3. Do you complete tasks in order?

4. Do you take pleasure in checking tasks off when they are accomplished?

5.   Are you good at spelling, grammar, and punctuation?

6.   Are you good at maths and following directions?

7.   Do you memorise words or mathematical formulae?

8.   Do you use information piece by piece to solve a problem?

9.   Do you look for pieces to draw a logical conclusion?

10.   Are you good at using words to give directions?

11.   Do you want to know the rules and follow them?

12.   Do you prefer information to be presented in a table?

Add up your yes answers. If you have mostly answered yes for the above questions, then you are more left brained than right brained. If you have only answered yes a few times, you are more right brained than left brained.

Action - Your Goals

Take some time now to make a list of the goals you would like to accomplish. Make sure that they are measureable i.e. how much and by when. Think about goals for some or all aspects of your life – could you write down all the goals that you want to achieve before you die? If you have created a Vision Board, you could use it to help you. Here are some areas for you to consider:

- Creativity
- Learning
- Family
- Friends
- Wellbeing
- Community
- Financial

Creativity – capturing your whispers

I invite you to use all or some of these prompts and record your responses in whatever creative way you choose.

- What are your passions?
- What are your dreams for your life?
- Where are they now?
- Where are you in your life?
- What is one thing you thought you could never do?

Enjoyment is about having fun along the way. Not worrying about what others may think, feel, say or do. It is about your nourishment. Do what you need to do today to bring Enjoyment into your life.

Chapter 4
THE MACE PATHWAY: ENJOYMENT

In 2010, if someone had asked me what I enjoyed, my honest answer would have been I don't know. My thoughts on enjoyment were that it was a waste of time, frivolous and unnecessary. My attitude was that I was far too busy and I had no time to be enjoying myself. However, deep underneath all of that negativity, I was longing for the day when I could enjoy myself, maybe have a holiday. I was putting my enjoyment, and with that my life, on hold for another day. I saw enjoyment as purposeless.

I saw my self-worth linked very much with work-worth, and that was cemented to levels of achievement at work. Using my time doing something purposeless just made me feel more anxious. I had so much to do and so little time to do it in. The thought of using up my time on something that was unrelated to my work or my to do list just created more anxiety and stress. There were times when I convinced myself that even sleeping was a waste of time. I had so much to do, and so little time. I had no time to fool around enjoying myself. I only had time to recover a little so that I could do more work-related jobs and things.

This attitude was pushing me into a dark, small and lonely hole. If I had understood that the opposite of enjoyment was this dark place, I probably would have included more enjoyment in my life. The MACE Pathway: ENJOYMENT, places enjoyment back into the centre of the arena of simple everyday activities, with every moment having the possibility to bring joy.

The MACE Pathway: ENJOYMENT is about acknowledging the special person that you are, opening and spreading your butterfly wings to have fun and joy along the way. Without joy or play life would be quite different. Imagine a life without books, without movies, art, music, jokes, personal stories, anecdotes and narrative. No daydreaming, no comedy, no irony. Such a world would be a pretty grim place to be. In a broad sense, enjoyment, play and fun, is what lifts us out of the mundane. I think enjoyment is like oxygen; it's all around us yet goes mostly unnoticed or unappreciated until it is missing. Talking and sharing with the participants on my workshops with colleagues and friends, I have come to understand that not knowing what we enjoy is quite commonplace and very much a part of the life many of us lead. This is particularly true if we are experiencing stress or putting our own life on hold for any reason. Having fun or enjoying ourselves almost becomes a guilty pleasure. Nearly every one of us starts out playing quite naturally. As children we don't need instruction in how to have fun. We just find what we enjoy and do it. We crave our individuality – our special selves. We want to be seen for the essence of who we are and enjoyment brings this close to us.

The MACE Pathway adopts the attitude that we all have our personal slant on what brings us enjoyment, but enjoying our moments is an essential component to The MACE Pathway. There is no right or wrong or good or bad way to enjoy. Exploring ourselves through fun and joy brings us closer to changing the way we see things now so we can have our time for freedom.

Balance and Wellbeing

Balance is a state of equilibrium that is essential to human beings. Yet our world around us is often out of balance, and it is for this reason that so many of us feel imbalanced. Constant change affects our lives through speed, uncertainty and new technologies. These all demand that our basic human needs are ignored.

Work life balance is traditionally interpreted as a balance between work and life as if there is always a clear divide between the two. Life balance is about feeling that we have our own freedom balanced with the discipline required to meet the demands and obligations we are facing. Finding the right balance in life can be a challenge for many of us. As much of our time and attention is focused on our work or our business, we may end up paying little or no attention to other areas in our lives. Life balance is about successfully and joyfully managing and living our lives. It is about balance between the extremes, between creativity and chaos, moving and stillness, work and leisure. It is about having a feeling of control over knowing when to shift from one to the other and being able to do so. Life balance, at its core, is about being balanced within, and feeling connected with ourselves and with our environment in a synchronised way.

Our points of balance are unique to us: each of us is slightly different from the other. I am constantly challenging myself and changing the way I see things now, and I am at my best when I am in balance. In Pathway Gems is a description of how to create your own Balance Wheel, which is a self-analysis of personal balance. I find completing this wheel three or four times a year helps me to keep a check on my own balance.

The MACE Pathway puts enjoyment and balance together, because when we have enjoyment in our lives we are creating balance. Balance is essential to our lives because it is a self-renewal process that we as human beings spread across all areas of our lives. In my workshops participants talk of wanting to create more life balance. When I have worked with children and young people, they are often trying to create more balance between study and fun. Balance makes our lives work well. When our lives are working well and we feel good about ourselves, we can be sure that we are in balance. You will always know when your life is out of balance because life begins to become difficult. And the opposite is also true: life is balanced when it feels like it is flowing.

Health

If you are unhealthy you will be unfocused and fatigued and stress will probably be running your life. Having a healthy strong life force that enables you to live your life with quality will mean that you can be more open to having fun, joy and play.

In 2010 I did not realise it but I was unhealthy. Apart from being stressed, in the previous five years I had pneumonia twice and swine flu once. I was seriously tired and the joints in my hips, knees and ankles ached often. I also had regular swelling in my ankles and feet. The tiredness I thought was linked to the stress, and the swelling and aches I put down to being old. My stressed emotional state led to a physical dysfunction that gradually led to a limiting in my understanding of what I actually enjoyed. I thought that once I finished teaching and had a rest I would be okay. I could not have been further from the truth. Six months from leaving teaching, although I was more relaxed, all my physical symptoms still existed.

This was until I met Dr GP McRostie OMD a health practitioner who lives in Aberfeldy, Scotland. After only two visits over six months my joints were no longer sore or stiff, the swelling in my ankles disappeared and I suddenly had more energy in my little finger than I had in my whole being six months earlier. One of the causes of this complete turnaround with my health is an omission of refined sugar and white flour from my diet.

Through my research and with Dr McRosties help, I found out about how sugars affect our bodies, our heart and blood vessels. When sugar levels are high in our bodies, insulin loses the ability to put glucose into our cells, so our metabolism loses its ability to give us energy. As a consequence glucose rises in our blood stream, our glands increase insulin production and the production of stress hormones, which in turn raises our blood pressure.

I thought that I had a healthy diet: vegetarian with very little sugar. However I have become aware of the hidden sugars in packaged food generally, not only desserts, snack foods and soft drinks, but also breads, packaged cereals, pizza, not to mention fruit juice. It is also useful to note that fructose and corn sweeteners are the worst as they require even less metabolising before flooding the blood stream. I was about to buy some ordinary organic nuts in an ordinary everyday supermarket, when I looked at the contents on the packet: it informed me that the nuts had been coated with corn syrup!

In nature, sugars are in a carbohydrate complex with many nutrients that protect our cardiovascular system, and require multiple metabolic processes before glucose can be utilised. I now eat more fruit for snacks and desserts, and read the labels on packaged food and am beginning to educate myself on this issue. Therefore my life force increases each day. I feel stronger, healthier and my clarity of thought grows daily.

Some information about vital nutrition

When we are living in a stressed and pressured way it affects our body's ability to assimilate nutrients. This can lead to a undernourished body, particularly with regards to hydration. When we are stressed our bodies go through a dehydration alert, which means cholesterol is secreted and coats each cell in order to protect the fluid inside. Once a cell has been coated in this way, it is difficult for the nutrients to enter it and toxins cannot easily leave. The result is a high level of acidity in your body. This in turn causes further stress. There are two rules that we can follow with our diet that helps keep our bodies healthy and protects us from harmful effects of stress:

Rule 1. Make sure that the acid-alkaline balance in your food is correct. That means that bodies need more:

- Fresh vegetables and fruit
- Sprouted seeds and herbs
- Cereal grasses
- Tofu and tempeh

And less acid forming foods, for example:

- Wheat and most grains
- Meat and fish
- Fast foods
- Cheese
- Sugar

Rule 2. Our bodies consist of approximately 75 per cent water. Water is vital in transporting nutrients throughout the body. As a result, its presence is essential in boosting energy levels and controlling body temperature, as well as the process of detoxification. Increasing your water intake and re-hydrating your body can quickly increase your resistance to stress; therefore, a regular intake of water throughout the day is best.

Being healthier has been a huge gift that I have given to myself. Somewhere in my thoughts I had a paradigm that I was living out, which told me that if I had aches and pains that was now a feature of my life because I was in my late fifties. And there was nothing I could do about it. Meeting Dr McRostie (albionbiologic.co.uk) challenged my paradigm and as a consequence I have got my life back.

Rest, relaxation and sleep for health

Through my experience, and talking to participants in my workshops, I began to see that enjoyment and rest are essential for our health. Enjoyment helps our brain to foster empathy, to work with social groups and complex situations, and at its root we can uncover the core of creativity. I also learnt about the importance of renewal through sleep, and through sleep came balance. Remembering that our bodies need rest and renewal so that they can give their best for the busy day ahead involves getting our sleep by going to bed as early as possible. Our systems, particularly the adrenals, do the majority of their recharging or recovering while we are asleep. Drinking relaxing herbal teas and avoiding caffeine late at night is very helpful, so is establishing a bedtime routine, which could include gentle yoga and meditation or relaxation. This all helps to clear the slate of the past day and prepare for the next. Plain lettuce is a natural sedative and the chlorophyll in green vegetables promotes sleep.

Relaxation is the state of wellbeing you experience when you stop creating tension, stress is the body's response to any change, whether pleasant or unpleasant. The secret is to manage this response so that rather than turning into negative stress, or distress, it energises you and acts as a springboard to empowerment.

There are 1,440 minutes in a day. You only need to achieve 20 of conscious relaxation. During those 20 minutes of relaxation you can clear the negative effects of stress. This is because an alpha brain wave state predominates in which your heart rhythm becomes more regular, your immune system is stimulated and can be improved, you feel at peace with yourself and your consciousness is being drawn away from external stimuli and functions at a deep level or awareness.

Yoga

The classical techniques of yoga date back more than 5,000 years. In ancient times, the desire for greater personal freedom, health and long life and heightened self-understanding gave birth to this system of physical and mental exercise, which has since spread throughout the world. The word yoga means, 'to join or yoke together' and it brings the body and mind together into one harmonious experience.

The whole system of yoga is built on three main structures: exercise, breathing, and meditation. The exercises of yoga are designed to put pressure on the glandular systems of the body, thereby increasing its efficiency and total health.

Yoga is helpful to the body for the following reasons:

- Stress Relief: The practice of yoga is well known for reducing the physical effects of stress on the body. The body responds to stress through a fight-or-flight response, which is a combination of the sympathetic nervous system and hormonal pathways activating and releasing cortisol, which is the stress hormone, from the adrenal glands. Cortisol is often used to measure the stress response. Yoga practice has been demonstrated to reduce the levels of cortisol.

- Better Breathing: Yoga includes breathing practices known as pranayama, which can be effective for reducing our stress response, improving lung function and encouraging relaxation. Many pranayamas emphasise slowing down and deepening the breath, which activates the body's parasympathetic system, or relaxation response. By changing our pattern of breathing, we can significantly affect our body's experience of and response to stress. This may be one of the most profound lessons we can learn from our yoga practice.

- Flexibility: Yoga can improve flexibility and mobility and increase range of motion. Over time the ligaments, tendons and muscles lengthen, increasing elasticity.

- Increased Strength: Yoga asana use every muscle in the body, increasing strength literally from head to toe. A regular yoga practice can also relieve muscular tension throughout the whole body.

- Improved circulation: Yoga helps to improve circulation by efficiently moving oxygenated blood to the body's cells.

- Presence: Yoga connects us with the present moment. The more we practise, the more aware we become of our surroundings and the world around us. It opens the way to improved concentration, co-ordination, reaction time and memory.

I explored many of the Yogic traditions before I settled with Dru Yoga. I developed my yoga practice through attending regular classes and then qualified as a yoga teacher. My yoga classes are open to middle aged and older people and are tailored to the level of the individuals. More information is available from my website. I wanted to manage my stress levels, physically strengthen my body, emotionally enhance my mind and bring some enjoyment into my life. Dru Yoga gave me the tools to take into my daily life and help me cope with much of the stress. Dru Yoga has its roots in Hatha Yoga, and includes classical yoga postures (asanas), pranayama (the science of breath) mudras (hand gestures), positive affirmations, empowering visualisations and powerful sequences performed in a flowing and dynamic style. For more information, please see Druworldwide.com.

Meditation

Meditation is the art of silencing the mind. When the mind is silent, concentration is increased and we experience inner calm in the midst of worldly turmoil. Stillness is what attracted me to meditation and I qualified as a Dru Meditation teacher. I meditate each day because I enjoy it. It may seem strange, but I feel happiest when sitting in perfect silence. The experience is difficult to express in words. It is also true that every meditation is not the same. Sometimes meditation is a struggle to control the mind, while at other times it feels effortless. When I first began to meditate, I was shocked to discover how unruly my mind was. Totally unconnected thoughts came and went at an amazing speed. Sometimes our minds feel like they will not settle, overwhelmed and submerged by a chaotic flood of images, memories and imaginings. Meditation is the journey from this unruly state to another kind of wilderness where I could focus on patiently calming those unruly forces. This journey is one of baby steps and takes time and energy. Little bit by little bit we get there. Some days are better than others. However all days are perfect because we are taking our steps towards cultivating a mind that's as spacious as a clear blue sky, as still as a lake at dawn, as stable as a mountain, and as full of subtle currents of energy as a forest full of wild creatures.

These are some of the benefits of meditation:

- Improved concentration: a clear mind makes you more

productive, especially in creative disciplines such as art, writing, etc.

• Less bothered by little things: do you sometimes allow yourself to get upset by little things? It is the nature of the mind to magnify small things into serious problems. Meditation helps us detach. We learn to live in the here and now, rather than worrying about the past or future. We do not worry about meaningless things, but see the bigger picture.

• Better health: there have been numerous studies pointing to the health benefits of meditation. The reason is that meditation reduces stress levels and alleviates anxiety. If we can reduce stress, many health benefits follow.

• Knowledge of self: meditation enables us to have a deeper understanding of our inner self. Through meditation we can gain a better understanding of our life's purpose.

As with yoga, I have followed the Dru Meditation tradition. Dru Meditation is about finding a still inner point from which you can look at the world in a different way and discover a fresh new perspective on your life. Using powerful breathing techniques (pranayama), and concentration techniques, you will learn to access a deep inner peace, no matter what challenges you might be facing. In Pathway Gems there is a short Meditation.

Walking

Walking is a magnificent synthesis of physical health, mental clarity and emotional freedom. It is perfect for creating a happy, balanced human being. One of the greatest gifts it provides is that of simplicity. When you walk, you cannot carry your furniture or your wardrobe. You only have yourself and your connection to nature.

Walking is an ordinary everyday activity that most people take for granted. Until I had swollen ankles and feet I certainly took it for granted. This small expression of my body's ill health ensured that I was unable to walk very far otherwise my feet hurt. Walking is also an excellent and free natural exercise that can help you stay healthy and live longer, control your weight, keep happy, enjoy time with friends and family, learn more about your local area and even look after the environment.

There are many benefits to walking. It generates health and vitality within the body through movement. Leg muscles are toned, feet are activated, and the spine is rocked. Deeper breathing is encouraged which cleanses the blood and calms the mind.

Doctors agree that regular physical activity like walking helps protect the body from many illnesses and conditions, including heart disease and stroke, high blood pressure, osteoarthritis, obesity, the most common type of diabetes and many cancers. It's also a great way to relieve stress and stay happy. Everyone knows how a good walk can help you collect your thoughts, and being outdoors, especially in green spaces can help fight depression and improve mental health.

And the best news is, almost everyone can do it, anywhere and at any time for free! You don't need special clothing, equipment or training and there are no gym memberships to pay. It's so easy and natural and there's very little risk you'll injure yourself.

Walking in nature allows us to absorb fresh energy. It is good to plan regular walks out of the urban environment, either each month or every other month. When we walk in nature it means that we are taking time out to gain perspective on our lives. Go alone or go with a companion and make sure you have fun along the way.

Celebrating personal stories

I am an ordinary person just like you. I am an expressive and sensitive woman who is always learning,. We are all connected, intertwining in this life. It is because I believe that we are all connected that I believe in the power and fun of sharing our stories. Those stories deep inside us: the stories about the ordinary, stories about courage, stories about change, short stories, long stories. All of our stories have importance, and sharing our stories as gifts is a special time of joy for everyone involved.

Do you know how interesting, powerful and unusual you are? Most of us don't There is a strong common belief that we are what we do. We also have this belief that other people have far more interesting stories to share. From talking to children, people that I have worked alongside and participants in my workshops, there seems to be a common agreement that many of us do not necessarily recognise the importance and value of our own stories. There is a real tendency to dismiss what is familiar without acknowledging that all our stories have power. Our stories begin when we arrived on this earth, and include all of our experiences. What scares us, what excites us and what fills us up. We are treasure chests waiting to burst open.

Our thought processes sometimes stand in the way of our stories through habits, old conditioning and memories. I record my stories mainly in writing and I use colour and shapes. I write about the good times and the bad times, I write it all. I write about my family, what I remember of the stories that my dad told me and descriptions of long gone friends and loved ones. I also write about what is boring me, how pathetic I feel at times as well as the brave feelings. Sometimes I even write about my double chin and how it is changing with age! When I am writing, I include my inner critic. Those words that are inside my head that are always very critical of what I am doing. I can't silence her so I include her. It is interesting to see her rantings and moanings appear on the page. I always remember that my stories are there to delight myself first.

Recording our stories by using pictures, drawings, colour or writing, I believe can be fun and can show us how wise, brave and human we are as well as helping us to remember who we are, that we are capable and loveable and significant and this creates connection and magic. Putting your story onto paper can be a visual journey, using, collage, pens and pencils. I sometimes use articles and visuals from magazines or photographs. I like experimenting with how I record and celebrate the everyday ebb and flow of my feelings about my life. Have some fun today. Get out your paper, pens, paint, and clay and begin to create and explore your stories and memories. The result is unimportant, what is important here is the risk and the fun.

Finding the beauty and truth in the ordinary.

Everything is special. In learning to look closely at the moments of our everyday lives, we find abundant inspiration that can spark our creative ideas and expression and we can begin to play. We can see for the first time the specialness of a stone, a leaf and sunset. We can now reach a far richer level of enjoyment. Everyday moments become clearer with meaning; sometimes they are moments that we have not noticed before. Our creativity just flows from paying closer attention to the abundance that already exists in the ordinary moments in our lives.

I have many ways of finding the beauty and truth in the ordinary; I take a photo, draw it, paint it or record it with words and pictures. This is about recording my everyday happenings of the small discoveries along the way of each of my days. Someday I will go for a short walk around the streets of east London and return hours later. Sometimes I record a sunset that reminds me of possibility and reminds me to use yellow, pinks, reds and oranges in my painting. Or I have recorded lampposts or doorsteps that remind me of my history and the beauty of distressed and used things. Sometimes I leave home with a shape in my mind, for example this can be circular, spiral and sometime heart shaped. I collect these shapes from what I see on my walk. They are representing small and meaningful speckles of universal loveliness and meaning. All of my collecting inspires me to think about how I express my creativity to the world. The colours I am drawn to and the colours I may use in the future to express my work. Each walk is an adventure into joy and in looking, paying attention and celebrating the beauty of the details of what is around me.

Creating community.

We all have a story as life in progress wanting to be heard; wanting to be seen, celebrated and lifted up. We are human beings, and sometimes we feel alone. Sometimes we struggle to find our place within the groups of people that we know. There is much enjoyment when you surround yourself with like-minded people. Kindred spirits. People who will be with you, side by side in a spirit of togetherness, without competition. Creative beings that will help you reach for the best parts of yourself and encourage you to fly. I believe that my friends contribute to my health and sanity and support me by telling and hearing the truth. I love them each dearly. I believe that the circles of friends around us weave invisible webs of love that support us, and nurture us when we feel down. They also sing and dance with us when we succeed and when we are strong. I invite you to lean back and rest in the arms of your friendships.

Giving

Giving and receiving is good for our health, wellbeing and brings us loads of fun!

A participant from one of my workshops shared the following story about receiving a smile. He wishes to remain anonymous.

'There was one day in the summer of 2010 – it was my worst day ever. I was stressed out and very unhappy. The next day was an important time in the school calendar and I needed to prepare for it. Things were not going too well at school and I was feeling very isolated. Even more reason that I managed the important event successfully. I was walking and the evening was heavy with a thunderstorm looming. I was carrying loads of papers and wanted to

get home before it rained, so they would not be ruined. A bus came along and I ran for it but it looked fairly full. People were elbowing their way past me to get on the bus and squeezing on. It seemed that this was the first bus for a while. Big spots of rain began to fall. I was desperate to get on the bus. As I put my foot onto the platform, the bus driver said that the bus was full and I could not get on. My heart sank and I pleaded with a young man who had the first seat to swap with me. He refused. As I turned around to leave the bus a young girl stood up and gave me her seat. She said that she was in no hurry and that she had a coat and an umbrella and didn't mind about the rain. I thanked her humbly and took her seat.

As the bus pulled away, I waved at the young women and smiled. And then I realised, that was the first time I had smiled all week. I had forgotten what it felt like. The muscles in my face felt relieved, I am sure. Tears welled up in my eyes. That one act of kindness made me realise how good kindness makes us feel.'

Kindness grows out of compassion and there have been suggestions that compassion could play a greater role in the maintenance of our good health. Gratitude is a mark of being kind to life by being aware of all that is around us, and when we are grateful, we acknowledge the people and situations in our life. Gratitude is also extremely health giving. Being grateful can make us happier and can improve the quality of our relationships.

Conclusion

I have shared my ways of creating enjoyment in my life. There is a wealth of possibilities out there, just waiting for you to dip in to. Enjoyment, fun and play comes in many flavours, colours shapes, sizes, tastes and sounds. Regardless of which one you like, it is important to enjoy your daily moments. I didn't always appreciate this. However, I when teaching and working with children I am reminded of the important role fun and enjoyment play in their lives, and most importantly to their learning. There is something very special about the way children get lost in the moment. Being carefree is at times a blessing. It allows you to be present instead of distracted. Have you ever wondered why time flies when you're having fun? It's because you have become so absorbed and immersed in what you're doing that you forget to look at your watch. You think only of the present without comparing it to the future or the past.

Children are great at having fun and being present and as adults, I think we have a lot to learn from them. We are overly concerned with the many other things in our lives while we are attempting to play. We have adult stuff on our minds. Getting in touch with what brings enjoyment into our moments will bring with it moments of magic.

Pathway Gems

Captured thoughts

'I hope you will go out and let stories happen to you, and that you will work them, water them with your sweat, tears and laughter till they bloom, till you yourself burst into bloom.'

Clarissa Pinkola Estes, author, poet and psychoanalyst

'I love people who make me laugh. I honestly think it's the thing I like most, to laugh. It cures a multitude of ills. It's probably the most important thing in a person.'

Audrey Hepburn, acress and humanitarian

Movement, Action, Creativity and Enjoyment

Movement – spinal wave

- With your feet hip-width apart, raise your arms sideways and up overhead as you breathe in.

- Fold forwards into a relaxed forward bend as you breathe out.

- Breathing in, slowly uncurl your body upwards, starting the movement from the base of your spine, with your head coming up last.

- As you return to the upright position, raise your arms sideways and up, stretching your entire body.

Repeat this spinal wave several times, moving slowly and with awareness of your spine unfolding in segments.

- As you uncurl upwards contract your lower abdominal muscles to assist with the extension of your spine.
- Keep your knees bent until your spine is nearly upright.

Action – Meditation

1. Relax for a few moments and focus on your breathing, watching the natural rhythm of each inhalation and exhalation.

2. Imagine a situation in your life that needs healing. Create an image of that situation in front of you, as if it were on a video screen. As you breathe in, draw some of the stress of the situation into your heart and immediately send it upwards and out of the top of your head as you breathe out. Feel that above your head is a region of golden light in which you have full access to your healing potential. Imagine the stress entering this region and visualise the situation being completely healed.

3. On an in-breath, draw this new situation into your heart and breathe it out into the scene in front of you, bringing peace and a good solution to that situation. See smiles of relief on the faces of everyone concerned.

Repeat steps 2-5 until you feel relaxed, calm and full of joy.

Action – The Balance Wheel

Wellness is all about maintaining a balance between different aspects of your life. Think of your life as if it were a wheel with eight spokes - if one spoke (one aspect of your life) is underdeveloped or neglected, the wheel (representing your overall wellness) will appear out of balance.

Everyone's representation of their optimal wellness is different. It depends on their own needs, experiences, personality, and circumstances. As we make our way through life, different aspects of life will fall in and out of balance, it's your job to try and maintain as much of a balance as possible in your life.

Now create your own Balance Wheel:

- Draw a circle to represent your life as a whole. This circle to be approximately 15 centimetres in diameter.
- Draw four lines rather like spokes in a wheel, within your circle. Creating eight even segments.
- Where all the lines cross in the middle of the circle put an even dot this represents zero.
- Each spoke radiates from the centre zero, to the out edge of the circle.
- Where each spoke reaches the outer edge of the circle write 10.
- In the middle of each spoke write 5.
- Each spoke from the centre to the out edge of the circle represents an area of your life, which is:
  1. Career/business
  2. Family/friends/community
  3. Finance
  4. Romance/partnership/marriage/intimacy
  5. Health/self-care
  6. Social/fun
  7. Personal/spiritual development
  8. Physical environment/home/office
- Write down what area of your life each spoke represents beginning with the top spoke and moving clockwise.
- Starting at the top spoke and moving around your wheel clockwise, give yourself a score between one and ten in the

different areas of your life indicated on your balance wheel. Only measure yourself against your own best, not anyone else's best. Carry out this exercise quickly listening intuitively to the first number that comes to your mind.

- When you have identified your individual scores, link the numbers. This will give you a picture of the balance of your life now. Life balance is always moving and tomorrow it could be different.

The aim is to have an even circle or wheel. If you have a dip then this maybe an area that you may want to focus your attention on.

Action – The Simple Things in Life

The MACE Pathway: ENJOYMENT is about bringing enjoyment into the simple things in our lives, which is essential if we want to bring about more joy. For your pure enjoyment you could carry out one or more of the following today.

- Smile at people you do not know.
- Describe yourself as gorgeous.
- Carry out random acts of kindness.
- Dress to please yourself.
- Let your creative spirit rush, flow, lead, spring, bubble out of you.
- End blaming.
- Tell the truth faster.
- Celebrate your gorgeous friendships.
- Discover yourself.
- Buy yourself a present.
- Take yourself on a walk for fun.
- Take risks and make mistakes.

- Share your uniqueness.

Action – The Kindness Challenge

Make a commitment to yourself that you are going to do an act of kindness each day for seven days. Some of these acts of kindness need to be anonymous – that means that no one can ever know that it was you who was kind. There is a list of possible acts, at the end of this chapter. Contact me via my website, elainemace.com and let me know how you get on.

Creativity – capturing your whispers

I invite you to use all or some of these prompts and record your responses in whatever creative way you choose.

- The questions I have about my journey are?
- Embracing my question, means?
- I don't need to know all the answers, because?
- When I feel the ebb and flow of my life, it means?

Enjoyment is about having fun along the way. Not worrying about what others may think, feel, say or do. It is about your nourishment. Do what you need to do today to bring Enjoyment into your life.

Ideas for Acts of Kindness:

1. Write a thank you card to someone.
2. Offer to carry a person's shopping, who needs it.
3. Allow someone in front of you in the supermarket checkout queue.
4. Give someone a compliment.
5. Buy an extra parking ticket and leave it on the parking meter

for the next person to find.

6. Pay for an extra pair of cinema tickets and ask the server to give them to someone they feel would appreciate them.

7. Leave £20 at the till of a local coffee shop and ask the manager to use it to pay for everyone's coffees until it is used up.

8. Tell someone in a shop or restaurant that they're doing a great job.

9. When someone cuts you up on the road, smile and wave at them.

10. Send a card to a teacher you once had and tell them how much they influenced your life.

11. Buy some food for a homeless person.

12. Use an online supermarket service and send a box of food to a family you know who could use it.

13. Join a charity as a regular volunteer.

14. Sing Happy Birthday to a friend on their birthday.

15. Offer your seat on the bus or train to a person who needs it.

16. Be a friend to someone in need.

17. Make a donation to charity.

18. Sponsor a child.

19. Buy a bag of apples or other fruit and hand them out on the street.

20. Make your loved one breakfast in bed.

21. Buy a gift for someone.

22. Buy lunch for someone who is short of money.

23. If someone is giving out leaflets in the street, take one and read it.

24. If you are ever given too much change, take it back to the shop.

25. Give blood.

26. Write a letter of gratitude to someone who has influenced your life.

27. If you are making tea for yourself make tea for everyone around you.

28. Send chocolates to a company that has given you a good service.

29. Send flowers to someone who enjoys them.

30. Find out what your friend really wants and provide it for them.

31. Buy a book for someone.

32. Offer to tidy a person's home/garden, who needs your help.

33. When a new person joins your work place, or into your street, make them feel welcome.

34. Hold a door open for someone.

35. Feed the birds.

Chapter 5

WHO IS SUPPORTING YOU ALONG YOUR PATHWAY?

The MACE Pathway is a commitment to change the way we see things, now. As The MACE Pathway spirals upwards, it enables us to collect the puzzles, the gems, the wisdom and the little pieces of our lives, to sort them out and create the most amazing and beautiful mosaic of our lives.

We may want to change the way we see things that relate to our work, our home, our relationships, or our life. Those first steps onto the pathway while focusing on where you are right now, and the attitudes that you wish to adopt, can feel like a risk because you do not know where they will take you. It is a step into the unknown. While treading the path and completing this work, you will make mistakes and you will learn. And that is fine. As the pathway spirals upwards, it will curve around your beautiful life, which will give you the opportunity to explore your viewpoints and give you the chance to create and commit to your goals. Enjoying your moments, breathing the air, absorbing the view, exploring ideas, enquiring, opening to curiosity and solving problems. Reaching the top of the mountain gives us the opportunity of having a panoramic bird's eye view of our life, welcoming all the questions that will inevitably bubble up, listening to them and considering possible answers is an essential part of The MACE Pathway.

Listening to our questions

Through creating and then applying The MACE Pathway to my own life, I brought movement, action, creativity and enjoyment into my life, and this inspired and empowered me to see things differently. This challenged the rigid way in which I was living my life. I became filled with questions that needed to be heard and that I needed to accept that I might not always know the answers to.

More than 30 years of teaching moulded me to live my life in a certain way. Mainly it taught me to manage my life as though it was lodged between two railway sleepers, firmly going in one direction with no space for flexibility or exploration. A long teaching career also taught me to be a taskmaster. It gave permission to my practical organisational nature to take over and micromanage all areas of my life. My life was a bundle of 'what ifs?' and 'shoulds.' There was no time for self-enquiry and questioning. Changing the way we see things now comes with a myriad of action questions, for example What should I do next? What exactly is my goal? Should I do it this way? So often we rush towards answers because not having a concrete resolution can make us anxious or worried. But the real truth is we so often sabotage our personal growth by providing a quick, swift answer to a question that is not yet ready to be answered. The MACE Pathway is not about quick answers or reaching a destination. It is about the journey that is often led by our questions, it is our life in the making. Following the MACE Pathway can feel like an adventure filled with the ebb and flow of life, filled with many questions. We often have questions and the answers may take time to surface. If we are making life-changing decisions and have questions that relate to circumstances the answers need time to permeate and to float to the surface.

I was going to leave teaching and take early retirement. I could have rushed at my decision. I felt anxious at the time, and a quick answer would have given me some relief, but may not have been a solution. When I have spoken about answering our internal questions in my workshops, some participants have talked about avoiding questions altogether. They feel that they have followed their paths without enquiry. Avoiding their internal questions led them to put their life on hold.

Keeping curiosity alive was a real motivator for me as a teacher, and I would do this through using open-ended questions and encouraging the children to do the same. Questions expand our inquisitiveness about our life. Our curiosity is our potential for growth. Ask open-ended questions to yourself: questions that do not have a right or wrong answer or a good or bad answer. Ask questions that you do not dare to ask. By asking them you may trigger or unearth the buried treasure of a hidden whisper. We may ask questions about our journey: What should I do next? Or more vague questions: What kind of person am I? Do I want to continue along this career path? How do I know that this is the right path for me? Sometimes knowing the answers to these types of questions is important, and sometimes the not knowing is equally important. What is important is to honour the questions that we have in our hearts, sit with them for a while, and nurture what it is they are trying to teach us.

Those internal questions do not need you to offer easy or quick solutions. They want to be heard and validated. The answers will come and will come later when you least expect them to, small moments unforced moments. It is the journey that matters after all; the journey along the mountain spiral of The MACE Pathway towards changing the way you see things now. The journey where our truth and answers breathe and dance. The MACE Pathway means being mindful of the opportunities that life has camouflaged in our unasked or unanswered questions. Maybe there isn't a next step right now. Maybe you don't have to know if you're on the right path at this very moment. Sometimes we have to sit with our questions without a task-orientated to do list or straight and narrow trail that leads directly to the answers. When we're doing what it is we're meant to do, when we allow our spirit a bit of freedom to roam the mysteries of the unknown, we can find our answers in the most unlikely places.

Nothing to lose by asking, but everything to possibly gain

Asking for support and making ourselves supportable is a strategy that creates focus so that we can change the way we see things. In my workshops, participants often share that they are resistant to asking for support. Most people it seems hold back by not asking for the information, money, time, or assistance that they may need to fulfil their vision and make their dreams come true. Mainly people do not ask for the support that they would like because they are afraid of looking silly, stupid, needy, and foolish. However sometimes underlying that is the fear of being rejected. That the person that they had chosen to help them might say no. Being afraid to ask for support and therefore not asking for support is actually saying no to ourselves. This behaviour makes sure that we have said no before anyone else has the chance to say it.

Some points to considering when asking for support:

- When asking for support, ask as if you expect to get it. Ask for whatever it is you want as though you already have received a positive answer. Ask as if you expect to get a yes.

- Before asking for support it is a good idea to consider what you are asking for, and to approach the person with a specific request. Be clear and specific. An example of an unspecific request for support:

  I asked a friend to proofread a draft of this book, and she said she would. I sent her the copy and did not hear again. I contacted her to ask what had happened and she told me that she had read it. And then she asked me if I wanted her to do something else with it. I had not been specific about my expectations with regards to proofreading. Therefore being clear and specific is very important in communication, and particularly when you are asking for support to make your dreams come true.

Your dreams are important so not giving up on them is vital. When you are asking for support you are asking another person to participate in your dream. This can make us feel vulnerable and reluctant to take a risk, just in case they say no. When we do ask our friends, colleagues or family for support, some of them may have other priorities, commitments and reasons not to participate in our dream The trick is to realise that they are not rejecting you; they are actually only saying no to your request. And to get clarity you can always ask why they have refused – this stops assumptions being made. However you could always return to them when they are in a different mood, on a different day, when you have new data or when the circumstances have changed. I think children have the best approach to asking and getting success. They will ask they same person for the same thing over and over again without any embarrassment at all!

Asking for what you want will move you forward into what's next. However for many of us, what holds us back from asking is the fear that we may be rejected. The MACE Pathway asks you to accept that some people will say no. It is inevitable that people will say no sometimes. However rejection is a myth. I was working on a gardening project in our communal garden and I wanted to put more logs in the garden. I sourced them and then when I had to move them around in the garden I decided to ask for support. I asked Debra, a neighbour, but she had to go to the shops and then I asked Morgan and he had to go to the park. The negative self-talk popped its head up and I quickly squashed it because I had begun this task alone, and actually, I was still alone. Nothing had changed. I was in the same situation that I was in at the beginning of the log project. I put my headphones in my ears, put on some music and began with my log moving. Debra returned from the shops with a mutual friend and they both helped me move the logs.

The truth is, there is never anything to lose by asking but everything to possibly gain. Getting stuck in fear and resentment will not move you along the pathway. By all means ask and remember that some will, some won't and so what! There are a lot of people on the planet – someone is waiting to say yes. And there is always someone out there who wants to be your Dream Keeper.

Who is your Dream Keeper?

During one of my workshops I was asked about what I had found to be the most important thing in maintaining conviction and dedication to my goals. I thought for a while, and replied 'my Dream Keeper'. Dream Keepers are those people who I completely confide in to help me to achieve my dreams. Dream Keepers come in many forms, Mentor, Coach, Dream Keeper Team, friends and colleagues. However they come into your life, Dream Keepers are there to support you, whether that's by listening, giving feedback, providing you with pots of tea or giving you their thoughts and ideas. What is really important about your dream keepers is that they are not there to compete, judge or criticise you or your dream.

Alexander Graham Bell had a Dream Keeper

Dr Alexander Graham Bell discovered the telephone with the help of his partner and Dream Keeper Thomas Watson. These two worked closely together while everyone at the time was dismissing them as odd and eccentric and wasting their time. One day, when Watson was working in another room to Bell, Bell had a serious accident and cried out for help. Watson was too far away to hear yet he did because Bell's cry was heard over the wires that the partnership was experimenting with. The rest of course is history.

Watson was Bell's Dream Keeper. We all need support to ensure that we keep moving in the direction we want to move in, and creating what we want to create in our world.

Finding your Dream Keeper

When we are working with our internal questions and looking for solutions, having a supportive community of Dream Keepers around creates clarity and empowers us to move forward towards our dreams.

When we are taking action towards our goals there are times are when we may experience our lives as a work in progress. These are times when sharing our story or celebrating our story can lift us up. Some of us welcome sharing with a group of like-minded people, knowing that a collective joy and connection can make us stronger.

The MACE Pathway is a journey, it may be a life-changing journey or it may be a smaller life problem needing a solution. However, it is good to surround yourself with people who are aware, tender and affirming. People who have a solid foundation within themselves to nurture you along your journey without competition. So choose your dream keeper carefully to ensure that they have the right qualities for you. If you can, choose someone who has already succeeded in something linked in some way to the path that you wish to travel. Choose wisely, who you share your dreams with. Stay strong and true to your goals and stand firm in your conviction and integrity!

Dream Keepers can come into our lives in many guises. Either as a Mentor, a Coach, a friend, or some people even have a Dream Keeper Team.

A Mentor

No matter where you are on your journey, you will more than likely have questions about your goals and your actions towards them. A mentor is an individual always more experienced in a similar field, who helps and guides another individual's development. This guidance is not done for personal gain. When I was teaching, my mentors were successful creative women who I met through my teaching career, and who were generous with their professional time and in answering my questions.

A Coach

I am fortunate enough that my Dream Keeper is also my coach. I have the greatest respect for someone who can not only guide and give sound advice, but also listen deeply. In all my interactions I feel valued, heard and most importantly empowered. Yes, I am definitely held accountable, so sometimes an email, sometimes a quick call or text, and I'm back on track. My coach is a kind of change agent. Goals, plans, new practices, achievements of every kind are all part of my work. My coach is an important element in the process of accelerating change. My coach guides me and listens to my bits and pieces about my journey as I stumble around my new life. She gives me practical advice, listens, and challenges me in ways my closest friends and family cannot.

A Friend

We all have people close to us who mean well. For them to be a good Dream Keeper it is a good idea to establish some ground rules first. This can be as simple as:

- Under no circumstances will you be negative about my goals.
- You will not share or gossip.
- You will listen to my ideas and help me develop them, even if at first they sound a little far-fetched.

This is to ensure that you have a trusting relationship, whereby you can share anything you want to without feeling in any way that you are not achieving your aims and goals, and also that you are able to reach for the stars if you so wish! This also means that when you aren't quite on track you can give them permission to hold you accountable for what you said you would do.

A Dream Keeper Team

Dream Keeper Team is a group of like-minded people who have separate and sometimes differing goals, co-operating together and supporting each other to successfully achieve their goals. A Dream Keeper Team can be made up of people in your social networks of colleagues or friends. You will probably be surprised at how willing many people are to help when asked, since it is an honour to be asked for advice or an opinion and to join a Dream Keeper Team.

- In my experience Dream Keeper Teams have formed around groups of adults, young people or children, who within their group are striving for a common purpose, whether that be about putting on a performance, improving fitness, taking retirement or creating a new beginning. The list is endless.

- Three to five people in each Dream Keeper Team is fine. This keeps meeting time short, in depth and on point. You can experiment with more or fewer, but I recommend starting with two or three if this is your first time working with a group in this way. Committed people working together with mutually committed partners creates a dynamic environment, that is the root of any Dream Keeper Team and each team has its own advantages:

  - Accountability: Members hold other members to account for the their goals.

  - Resources: Everyone in a team comes with access to a different skillset and network of people.

  - Differing perspectives: All members see issues from different points of view, whether they are agreed with or not. Hearing another's point of view always gives a better understanding of what is possible.

I offer some ground rules about how to run a Dream Keeper Team in the Action section, in Pathway Gems at the end of the chapter.

Feed forward or Feedback?

When we ask questions of our supportive and empowering community of Dream Keepers, there will inevitably be feedback. Advice, help, data, suggestions, direction and criticism will help you to adjust and move forward, and at the same time enhance your knowledge, skills, attitudes, understanding and relationships.

There are two kinds of feedback, negative and positive. Most of us prefer positive feedback. Feedback that tells us, that we are doing the right thing and *en route* to getting where we want to be. Negative feedback tends to tell us that we are headed in the wrong direction or doing the wrong thing. However, it is also very valuable information for our learning. In my workshops, I talk about how important it is to take risks, make mistakes and that it is only then then that we are able to learn and grow. Mistakes are inevitable, and therefore feedback that tells us that we are going in the wrong direction is welcomed. All feedback helps us decide how to get back onto our desired pathway and towards our dream. Some people who have attended my workshops have found focusing on changing how they see negative feedback helpful. Changing the way I see things has helped me reframe negative feedback to an improvement possibility. Negative feedback is the world giving me valuable information that will enable me to correct and improve what I am doing so that I can achieve my dream. To reach my goal or dream quickly, I welcome, receive and embrace all the feedback that comes my way.

It is important to learn how to respond to feedback. There are some responses that do not help you towards your growth:

- Ignoring the feedback when listening to feedback could be supportive. Not listening means that you could be ignoring something that could potentially significantly transform your life.

- Getting mad at the person who is giving the feedback. Getting angry with the person, who is giving you feedback, will only push them away. You could be pushing away someone that could potentially and seriously transform your life.

- Crying and giving up. If you cry and give up when you receive feedback, all this will do is keep you in the same place. And the person who is giving you feedback will be reluctant to give you feedback in the future. You could be pushing away someone that can help transform your life.

Feedback is guidance and not criticism. It will help you grow and improve, and create movement, action, creativity, and enjoyment towards your goal. Think of an automatic pilot system on an aeroplane. The system is constantly telling the plane that it is either too high, too low, too far to the right or too far to the left. The aeroplane keeps correcting in response to the feedback it receives – it does not become emotional (thank goodness!). Feedback is information designed to help you adjust and take action towards your goals and dreams.

Passion and enthusiasm

Passion and enthusiasm are two words that very much go together. Passion is something within us that provides us with the continual enthusiasm, drive, attitude, and confidence needed to succeed. But unlike feel-good motivation derived from external sources, true passion has a more internal or spiritual nature. It comes from within, and can be channelled and focused. There are people from history and from our own lives who we know of as passionate.

Passionate people are all around us, those people who are enthusiastic about their work, their garden, their children, their hobbies, their cooking, and their love of life. They cannot wait to get up in the morning and get started. Passionate people are eager and energetic. They are filled with purpose and committed to their lives. This kind of passion comes from enjoying and loving your work. It comes from doing what you were born to do. It comes from following your heart and trusting your joy as a guide. Enthusiasm and passion come as a result of caring about what you do, discovering your true purpose and deciding what you really want to do and have and believing that you can do and have it.

139

Conclusion

One of the realities that I have learned about life is that changing the way we see things now takes time and a commitment to constant improvement. Changing and improving takes time. It does not happen overnight. We live in a speedy culture where there is an expectation that gratification will be instant. We can become discouraged when it doesn't happen. However if you make a commitment to walk the MACE Pathway each day eventually over time you will reach your goal.

Leading your own life into the direction you want it to go takes time. You have to practise and focus your skills through refinement and constant use. It takes years to produce expertise, insight and wisdom. Every book you read, every class you take, and every experience you have is another step towards your goal and along the MACE Pathway. Being ready for what's next is important. Don't short-change yourself by not being ready when something you have always wanted appears in your life.

As a teacher, I was constantly returning to the classroom to learn new teaching and learning strategies. In the area of personal development I am constantly reading new material, researching new ideas, and attending talks, workshops and courses to expand my knowledge and to ensure that I am constantly improving. I am always engaged in a process of improvement. Artists explore new mediums, doctors learn about new procedures, writers read about new ways of creating a plot. Making a commitment today to improve in every way will enable you to enjoy the feelings of increased self-esteem and self- confidence that comes from self-improvement, as well as the success as you move ever closer towards your goal.

Pathway Gems

Captured Thoughts

'The purpose of relationships is not to have another who might complete you: but to have another with whom you might share your completeness.'

Neal Donald Walsch, Author

'My friends have made the story of my life.'

Helen Keller, Author, political activist and lecturer

Movement, Action, Creativity and Enjoyment

Movement – deep yogic breath technique

Breathing is not only one of your basic survival skills, it is also one of your most powerful and accessible tools for improving your mood and regulating your metabolism.

You can calm panic, lift depression, slow a racing heart and more just by changing your breathing pattern. Yet most of us have never been taught how to breathe.

Please note: changing your breathing cycle can be a powerful practice so be aware of the feelings in your mind and body. If you begin to feel any unpleasant sensations, such as tingles, light-headedness or giddiness, return to normal breathing, lie down on your stomach or go and do something soothing and relaxing. Always listen to the limits of your own body. If you have a heart condition or blood pressure issues please check with a medical practitioner.

How to do the deep yogic breath.

1. Either sit on a chair or lie comfortably on the floor. If sitting, ensure that your feet are flat on the floor, your lower legs are at right angles with your thighs and your thighs at right angles with your back. Also try placing a cushion under the rear of your buttocks to ensure the pelvis is tilted slightly forward to give a slight arch in the lower back.

2. Engage core stability muscles and take a few breaths to allow your body to relax and your gaze to soften.

3. When ready, focus your attention on your diaphragm, the muscle that controls breathing.

4. Allow your diaphragm to slowly expand down into the abdomen and as you do this, notice your lungs filling with air. Contract the diaphragm and the breath leaves the lungs.

5. Repeat this a few times and you may already notice a different in your mind and body.

6. Once you are comfortable with this breathing pattern, become aware of the bottom third of your lungs and breathe into and out of this part of your lungs for a few breaths.

7. Now become aware of the middle section of your lungs and on your next breath, breathe into the bottom then the middle of your lungs (around heart level, otherwise called thoracic) then breathe out from the bottom then middle. Repeat for a few breaths.

8. Finally, become aware of the very top section of your lungs and breathe into the bottom, middle then top section of your lungs. Allow the air to fill to the collarbones, exhale, again by contracting the diaphragm, from the bottom, middle and then top of your lungs. Repeat this no more than 10 times in a session to begin with and gradually build into a longer practise.

9. Allow your body to relax slowly into this breathing pattern, never straining or breathing to your full capacity.

10. Take a few moments to ease back into normal breathing and notice how you feel.

Action – Take Five Steps Towards Your Goal Today!

If each day you were to take five steps towards your goal then eventually, no matter how long your pathway was, you would reach the end. I use this metaphor to illustrate the fact that if we take five steps towards our goal each day, at some point we will reach our goal, no matter how small our steps are.

What are your five steps today?

Action – Dream Keeper Team Organisation

1. Meet regularly. It is essential to meet regularly and try not to move your meeting time around. I suggest 60 minutes per week.

2. Meet precisely.

   - Punctuality is essential.

   - End on time.

   - Three members to a team and 20 minutes for each member.

   - One person speaks at a time, no interruptions.

   - Hold comments until person has completed speaking.

   - No one jumps in, unless they have a very important question.

3. My Dream Keeper Team does not always have an agenda, sometimes we have a talk topic that would have been agreed at the previous meeting.

An agenda is useful for accountability and progress reports. Find out what suits your needs.

4. Do you need a team facilitator? When a group is starting out they sometimes need a person to hold the group, keep people on target for time, move on from agenda items etc.

5. Capture what happens at each meeting: successes, celebrations, goals, and items to keep others accountable too.

6. Questions to get your Dream Keeper Team up and running:

   • What are you working on?

   • What did you learn?

   • What do you need help with?

7. What's next?

Creativity – capturing your whispers

I invite you to use all or some of these prompts and record your responses in whatever creative way you choose.

Sit down in a quiet space and record all the things that you would like in your life, that you would like to ask for but that you do not. It might be at work, at home, or leisure. It might be to get some time off, a massage, a hug, help with a project, feedback or a loan. Next to each one, record what stops you from asking for what you want. And think about how are you losing out, because you do not ask and what the benefits would be from asking. Take time with your captured whisper, and consider what's next for you.

Enjoyment is about having fun along the way. Not worrying about what others may think, feel, say or do. It is about your nourishment. Do what you need to do today to bring Enjoyment into your life.

Chapter 6

FINAL WORDS

Throughout my life, I have often put myself through endless difficulties to avoid and escape life's challenges. At times, I tried to run away. Or look for someone to rescue me. The experience taught me many things: one of my greatest realisations was, what if this struggle is serving some purpose for me?

I found an interesting story recently, one that stimulated some deep thinking on this very question.

An Interesting Metaphor

A man found a butterfly cocoon. He took it home and placed it on the kitchen windowsill, where he could keep an eye on it. One day a small opening appeared. Curious, the man sat down at the kitchen table to watch. The cocoon began to move. The insect was beginning to push through the hole. For several hours it struggled to force its body through the tiny opening. Then all progress seemed to stop. It appeared that the butterfly could get no further.

So the man decided to help. With a pair of scissors, he made a slit to enlarge the hole.

Soon the butterfly emerged. Its body was swollen and its wings, small and shrivelled.

The man waited, sure that the wings would gradually enlarge and expand to support the body, as the body reduced to normal size.

Neither happened! In fact, the butterfly spent the rest of its life on the windowsill, flapping its under-developed wings and dragging its distended body around. It was never able to fly.

In his well-intentioned desire to be kind, the man did not understand that the restriction of the cocoon and the struggle required for the butterfly to get through the tiny opening was nature's way of pressing fluid from the body of the butterfly into its wings. The process was designed to perfect the butterfly's beauty and prepare it to fly in freedom, as soon as it left the cocoon.

Anonymous.

From this story I learnt that sometimes our struggles are exactly what we need at certain points in life. Without them, we might not develop the strength or skills or understanding we need to develop the wings that will take us to the heights of our destiny and allow us to 'fly' onto our next stage. As I progressed towards my sixtieth year, I needed to accept that I was outgrowing the life I had been used to but I was scared. I did not know who I was becoming and I did not know what life had in store for me. Once I understood that the process I was undergoing was a natural one, I started to relax and let it take its course and my life evolved into its next phase. Treaders of The MACE Pathway have much to learn from the butterfly cocoon story.

From Caterpillar to Cocoon: A caterpillar is a small fat furry larva that through metamorphosis becomes a butterfly. The metamorphosis takes place in the cocoon. Seek safety and be patient in your cocoon stage. You may be in a process of transformation for some time. Surround yourself with friends and family members you trust. Be kind to yourself through this transition. Remember your cocoon is temporary and the cocoon is a space that allows us to go through a major transformation. Hold onto your dreams and remember that:

- **What other people think of you is not your business.** Stop trying so hard to be something that you're not just to make others like you. It doesn't work this way. The moment you stop trying so hard to be something that you're not, the moment you take off all your masks, the moment you accept and embrace the real you, you will find people will be drawn to you effortlessly. Do whatever feels right for you, regardless of what other people have to say about it. Celebrate your authenticity.

- **It is okay to be alone.** To listen to our internal whispers sometimes we need to step back and re-evaluate a situation, a relationship or just life in general. When I left teaching, I took myself on an eight-day silent retreat organised by Dru Yoga. I wanted to become my own best friend again.

- **Change is inevitable.** Change is a factor you can be sure of. Change is good. Change will help you move from A to B. Change will help you make improvements in your life and also the lives of those around you. Follow your bliss, embrace change – don't resist it.

- **Decide on what you want to create in this world.** Decide on what is important to you and what you want to create in this world and take small steps towards it daily.

- **Self-talk will keep you small**. How many people are hurting themselves because of their negative, polluted, and repetitive self-defeating mind-set? Don't believe everything that your mind is telling you – especially if it's negative and self-defeating. You are better than that.

- **You are OK.** Give up your limiting beliefs about what you can or cannot do, about what is possible or impossible. From now on, you are no longer going to allow your limiting beliefs to keep you stuck in the wrong place. All of us have had times in our lives where we have thought, I'm not good enough or I am not the right weight or size. Give yourself a chance and spread your wings and fly!

- **The process is important.**
  Don't sabotage the process by making unwarranted assumptions. The man watching the butterfly in the cocoon thought he was helping, but was he? From our limited human perspective, we cannot always see the complete picture. It is tempting to jump to conclusions about what should or should not happen, what something does or does not mean, how long a stage should last or what progress should look like.

- **Keep your eye on what is important to your life.**
  When something goes wrong in our life, we can begin to pull our hair out and become miserable. A good question to ask yourself is what things are not going quite according to your plan and what is important right now? Give up on your need to blame others for what you have or don't have, for what you feel or don't feel. Stop giving your powers away and start taking responsibility for your life.

- **Give up criticising, comparing and complaining.**
  Give up your constant need to complain about those many things – people, situations, events that make you unhappy, sad, and depressed. Nobody can make you unhappy, no situation can make you sad or miserable unless you allow it to. It's not the situation that triggers those feelings in you, but how you choose to look at it. Never underestimate the power of positive thinking. We are all different, yet we are all

the same. We all want to be happy, we all want to love and be loved and we all want to be understood.

- **Face your fear and tell it that it has no place in your life.**
  Fear is just an illusion, it doesn't exist – you created it. It's all in your mind. Correct the inside and the outside will fall into place.

- **Acknowledge your personal progress.**
  Look closely. You are developing, growing, changing. Your wings are forming. Embrace the personal transformation that comes with the challenges, especially those that feel like a time of death and rebirth. In the words of Maya Angelou, 'We delight in the beauty of the butterfly, but rarely admit the changes it has gone through to achieve that beauty.'

- **Accept that you want to be happy.**
  There are so many of us who can't stand the idea of being wrong – wanting to always be right – even at the risk of being sad. It's just not worth it. Whenever you feel the 'urgent' need to jump into a fight over who is right and who is wrong, ask yourself this question: 'Would I rather be right, or would I rather be happy?' Wanting to be right means someone is wrong and that is how conflict is created in relationships and ultimately in the world. I would rather be happy creates far more win/win!

- **Allow yourself to feel what you feel.**
  Metamorphosis is intense and can be a highly emotional time. Bring your deep, heartfelt emotions up to the surface. Do not ignore them. Own them and honour them. By experiencing them honestly, you learn that you are bigger than these emotions. If you allow them to run their course, they pass, leaving a space into which peace can flow.

- **It's too late for excuses.**
  Send them packing and tell them they're fired. You no longer need them. A lot of times we limit ourselves because of the many excuses we use. Instead of growing and working on improving ourselves and our lives, we get stuck, lying to ourselves and using all kind of excuses – excuses that 99.9 per cent of the time are not even real.

- **Live in the present.**
  Be present in everything you do and enjoy life. After all life is a journey not a destination. Have a clear vision for the future, prepare yourself, but always be present in the now. Take everything one day at a time.

- **Live your own life.**
  Way too many people are living a life that is not theirs to live. They live their lives according to what others think is best for them, ignoring their inner voice, that inner calling. They are so busy with pleasing everybody, with living up to other people's expectations, that they lose control over their lives. They forget what makes them happy, what they want, what they need. And eventually they forget about themselves. You have one life – this one right now – you must live it, own it, and don't let other people's opinions distract you from your path.

The butterfly emerges

I think the metaphor of the life cycle of a butterfly is an interesting one to use when considering our own lives. At the end of the cycle it is not easy for the butterfly to break out of the cocoon. The butterfly alone has to fight and fight hard, to emerge. There is a purpose to its struggle as through this process it gradually gathers the strength and all that it needs to eventually fly and be a successful butterfly. It is good to remember that:

- **You are a human being and not a human doing.**
  You will make mistakes. You won't always feel happy and positive and that is okay. The next time you begin to give yourself a hard time over these things, remind yourself that you are imperfect and that you love, trust and believe in yourself.

- **Your story.**
  Remember to gift the world with your stories, words, drawings and doodles.

- **Creativity.**
  Creativity is in us all; it's the spark that lights us up. The important step to take is to begin.

Conclusion

I would like to encourage you to read this book twice. Make jottings either in your journal or in the margin about what is most important to you. Give yourself time to absorb The MACE Pathway. The ideas behind and underpinning The MACE Pathway are not new, in fact many of them are so old they are universal, and that is their ancient beauty. Share the ideas with the people close to you, help them understand and become free from their limiting beliefs, and empower them to set goals and hear their own call to action. We all have the power within us to create the life we want, the life we dream about, the life we were born to live. We all deserve to fulfil our dreams. We can claim this birth right but it will come through hard work and focus.

What if we all gave up complaining and took full responsibility for our lives and ourselves, and started creating the lives of our dreams? Can you imagine a world where everyone took 100 per cent responsibility for their lives and the results they create or do not create? A world that works for everyone with no one left out. Women, men and children would create collectives and community. People would ask for what they need and want. Another might

Butterfly, by Jana Stanfield / Joyce Rouse

Sitting alone on a hillside, confused about what to do.

My choices were all complicated, it was time to think
things through.

Spotted a striped caterpillar, stretching her face to the sky.

Dragging her cumbersome body an inch at a time.

I was feeling the pain of slow progress, when a friend of hers
fluttered by.

I leaned close as the caterpillar spoke with a voice
as soft as a sigh.

She said…

'Butterfly, please tell me again it's gonna be alright.

I can feel a change is coming.

I can feel it in my skin.

I can feel myself outgrowing

this life I've been living in.

And I'm afraid, afraid of change.

Butterfly, please tell me again I'm gonna be all right.

I'm like my friend caterpillar, afraid of that dark cocoon.

Wanting to hide in the tall grass, when change is coming soon.

But all of the things we long for are borne
on the wings of change.

And losses can lead us to blessings that we can't explain.

Butterflies remind us, there's magic in every life.

And we can become what we dream of,
if fat furry worms can fly.

answer no when the time was not right for them. Others might say yes. People would be busy creating the life that they want. People would tell the truth, listen to each other and be compassionate to others and themselves. In this world, peace, joy and abundance for all would flourish.

The greatest gift we can give to the world I believe is to love trust and believe in ourselves. And through our own self-awareness and self-realisation we will create win/win situations and therefore peace into our world. Someone has to start, is that going to be you?

Pathway Gems

Captured Thoughts

'How does one become a butterfly? You must want to fly so much, you want to give up being a caterpillar.'

Trina Paulus, Author

'There is a crack in everything, that is how the light gets in.'

Leonard Cohen, Singer/songwriter, author and poet

Movement, Action, Creativity and Enjoyment

Movement – Dance!

Play your very favourite dance music and move your body. You are on your own, no one is watching so have fun, and enjoy your time.

Action – Starfish Story

I would like you to imagine a beautiful wide golden sandy beach that stretches for miles. The warm crystal clear sea is lapping gently to the shore. Ways over to the right are some cafés surrounded by magnificent palm trees that are swaying in the gentle breeze.

Walking along the water's edge is a young woman. She is bending down and picking something up and throwing it into the sea. As she lets it go she is saying something.

A young man is also walking along the beach. He looks down and notices that around his feet are starfish. As his gaze rises, he sees that there are starfish as far as his eyes can see. Up to the cafés and back to the seashore. He notices the young woman and wonders what she is doing. He walks up to her and watches and listens.

The young man notices that the young woman is picking up the starfish and throwing them back into the sea. He taps the young woman on the shoulder and says to her 'Why are you bothering? You will never clear this beach of starfish! If you stay here all day and all night, it will still be covered with starfish. What is the point?'

The young woman listens to the young man. She bends down, picks up a starfish, and throws it into the sea. As she lets go of the starfish she points to where it lands in the water and she says 'I made a difference to that one.'

What action are you taking today, to make a difference?

Creativity – capturing your whispers

I invite you to use all or some of these prompts and record your responses in whatever creative way you choose.

Your prompt is this beautiful song from the singer/songwriter Jana Stanfield. The words resonate with me deeply and it always gives me a leg up into the fast lane of being over sixty!

If I Were Brave, by Jana Stanfield

What would I do if I knew that I could not fail?

If I believed, would the wind always fill up my sail?

How far would I go?

What could I achieve, trusting the hero in me?

If I were brave, I'd walk the razor's edge, where fools and dreamers dare to tread.

I'd never lose faith, even when losing my way.

What step would I take today, if I were brave?

What would I do today, if I were brave? What would I do today if I were brave?

What if we're all meant to do what we secretly dream?

What would you ask if you knew you could have anything?

Like the mighty oak sleeps, in the heart of a seed, are there miracles in you and me?

If I were brave, I'd walk the razor's edge, where fools and dreamers dare to tread.

I'd never lose faith, even when losing my way.

What step would I take today, if I were brave?

What would I do today, if I were brave? What would I do today if, I were brave?

If I refuse to listen to the voice of fear, would the voice of courage whisper in my ear?

If I were brave, I'd walk the razor's edge, where fools and dreamers dare to tread.

I'd never lose faith, even when losing my way.

What step would I take today, if I were brave?

What would I do today if I were brave?

Write, draw or doodle: what would you do today if you knew you could not fail?

Enjoyment – here's something you can do today. Have you ever felt that you wanted to make the world a better place? But stopped because you felt that it was completely beyond your reach?

Here is something you could do each day that will gently roll out your potential.

- As you prepare for bed, look back over the day.

- Make a list of those moments when you could have improved someone's life but you hesitated or resisted.

- For each moment envisage what you could have done and jot down ideas for action.

- For each idea ask yourself the following questions:

  - What great benefits would this action have brought to me, to the people around me and to all of life around me?

  - Write down your answers to these questions and in the morning look over your list again.

Repeat this process every day for 10 days and soon you will find that you will not be able to resist acting on more and more of these opportunities.

You will have begun to realise the power of your potential for making peace a reality around you. Imagine if you taught this simple but power practice to 10 people and they then taught it to another 10 and another ten?

END THOUGHTS FOR THE READER

Dear Reader,

Throughout my life, like you I have gained a wealth of knowledge, understanding, skills, and wisdom from a variety of life experiences. My experiences were collected from my personal life, from my world of work in teaching, and personal leadership. I began by working in Woolworths in the 1960s and retired as a primary school teacher in 2011 and I am now on the brink of something completely new. Throughout my life, I have dealt with the various things that life can throw at all of us.

I believe that we are all special, amazing, loveable, unique, blessed, brave and good enough human beings, with abundant amounts of love, wisdom, courage, stamina and strength. I also believe that we want to make a difference but sometimes our lives prevent us doing this. Creating the MACE Pathway supported me in unearthing my purpose, which is to inspire and empower children, women and men to love, trust and believe in themselves, so that they change the way they see things now and can create their best life. I developed The MACE Pathway to support me while I struggled with my own mid-life issues, although I am experienced and knowledgeable about personal leadership. As I lived and worked my way towards my sixtieth birthday, my life was thrown into turmoil. Creating The MACE Pathway gave me the structure that I needed to change the way I saw things and create my best life.

For many of us, when we reach mid-life we realise that some of our life has been on hold. The MACE Pathway can be used to blow the dust off our dreams, our passion, our loves, and our goals. The MACE Pathway takes this one step further and suggests movement, action, creativity and enjoyment is the secret of manifesting those dreams.

I will admit that I continue to be in the process of discovery about loving, trusting and believing in myself so that I can change the way I see things now. I believe deeply in sharing my ongoing story, because we all have a story to share. I am excited to share what I have discovered here in *The Time for Freedom*, and look forward to learning what I still don't know.

I would like *The Time for Freedom* to be an active companion on your journey in changing the way you see things now. A kind wise friend who tells you that you are good enough.

If you think that I could support you on your journey, or if you would like more information about my work, then please contact me at elaine@elainemace.com or via my web site at elainemace.com.

Best Wishes

Elaine Mace

BIBLIOGRAPHY & RECOMMENDED READING

Atavar, Michael, *How to be an Artist*, Kiosk Publishing, 2012

Brown, Brene, *The Gifts of Imperfection*, Hazelden, 2010

Cameron, Julia, *The Artist's Way*, Putnam, 2002

Coelho, Paulo, *The Alchemist*, HarperCollins, 1991

Dru Yoga, *Stillness in Motion*, Dru, 2005

Mark Victor Hansen & Robert Allen, *The One Minute Millionaire*, Vermilion, 2002

Mayne, Brian, *Goal Mapping The Practical Workbook*, Watkins, 2010

Mayne, Brian, *Sam The Magic Genie*, Vermilion, 2003

Pantanjali, *The Yoga Sutras of Patanjali*, Bell Tower, 1982

Patel, Mansukh, *The Freedom of the Bhagavad Gita*, Life Foundation Publications, 2009

Paulus, Trina, *Hope for the Flowers*, Paulist Press, 1972

Sark, *Succulent Wild Women*, Prentice Hall, 1997

Satir, Virginia, *Self Esteem*, Celestial Arts, 1975

All authors have websites

ABOUT THE AUTHOR

Elaine Mace is a passionate woman who has devoted much of the past 30 years to inspiring and empowering children, women and men to love, trust and believe in themselves. She is a prominent and experienced speaker, author, teacher, trainer and coach. The key design principles for Elaine's work are risk, creativity, honesty and flexibility. Using these principles she delivers powerful workshops, seminars, and training for children, teens and adults to build their self-confidence and self-worth. Elaine also provides insightful Personal Leadership Coaching, underpinned by The MACE Pathway.

If you think that Elaine could support you on your journey, or if you want to get more information about her work, then please contact her at elaine@elainemace.com or via her web site at elainemace.com

'I believe that we are all special, loveable, amazing, brave human beings, full of love, light, wisdom, courage, stamina and strength. I also believe that we want to make a difference but sometimes our lives stop us. My purpose is to inspire and empower children women and men, to love trust and believe in themselves, so that they change the way they see things now and create their best life.'

Elaine Mace, 2012

14312216R00096

Made in the USA
Charleston, SC
04 September 2012